Deepening The Power
Community & Sacred Theatre
by Celu Amberstone
Cornwoman

I0155379

Deepening the Power: Community Ritual and Sacred Theatre

Rituals, Volume 2

Celu Amberstone

Published by Kashallan Press, 2022.

DEEPENING THE POWER: COMMUNITY RITUAL AND SACRED THEATRE

First edition. June 30, 2022.

Copyright © 2022 Celu Amberstone.

ISBN: 978-1990581021

Written by Celu Amberstone.

Table of Contents

April 2022

A note to the reader:

This book was originally published in 1994. As I read through the manuscript again for this recent republication I found there wasn't much I wished to add to or change. What is written here is a culmination of much that I've learned over the 75 years of my life. It is my legacy, sort to speak, for those who will come after me. I hope it will be of use as a guide in our troubled world. With blessings and love I offer you this book, dear reader

Celu Amberstone (Cornwoman)

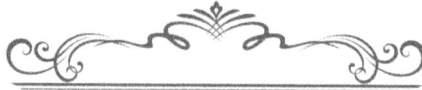

Preface

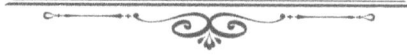

This book is drawn from my experience as a teacher and a practicing Pagan ceremonialist. In these pages I have tried to take all the bits and pieces of my technique and organize the material into a workable format for my students and others wishing to explore ritual and theatre within the community context. There are some outlines for the ritual processes in this book, but the aim here is not to instruct the beginner. There are several good books on the market that offer such instruction. It is my hope that this work will offer new perspectives and information to the already-practicing Pagan ceremonialist.

The reader may note that my approach to ritual and ceremony is somewhat different than most materials that have been written on the subject in the past few years. I attribute this difference to the training I received as a young woman from my Native and European elders. For more than fifty years I have studied in these ancient traditions. My training was strict and often hard. When I was younger I often felt limited and confined by these traditions. As I grew older and experienced rituals in other contexts such as the New Age Pagan movement, I began to realize what a wonderful gift I had been given when young.

The focus in these pages is on community ceremonials in all their pageantry rather than on personal devotions. I hope to offer some information and insights that will help us to recreate what was almost totally destroyed by Christian imperialism in the past.

Towards this end I offer in Part One a variety of loosely connected ideas and information that will help the reader see the difference between where we are now and what was there before. My purpose is not to criticize but to show what we need to reclaim from tradition to help us go on to the next step, which is, for me, building effective ceremonial practices for the future.

In Part Two, I discuss in more detail the actual community ceremonial process that I use when teaching ceremony to groups wishing to form that bond. The steps laid out will take some effort on the part of the group, but the rewards are more than worth it. As some of my students have pointed out to me, once they have experienced the power and beauty of these rites they have been spoiled for anything less.

In traditional societies around the world, one of the main reasons ceremony has such a powerful impact on the participant and observer is its use of sacred theatre. In doing research for this book I could find little written on this topic for the reader to use in designing modern ceremonials.

So, I offer in some detail what I have learned from other teachers and have developed myself. I hope this will inspire others to explore the use of theatre further in their ceremonial craft.

At present my teachings offer a flavor of Native North America, while the bulk of the content is European. I like to think of my style as a hybrid combining both aspects of my heritage, as well as paying homage to the spirits of the land upon which I live. It is my sincere belief that for most of us there is no real way to go back to the past. We all are hybrids of some type or other, and we need to recognize that fact and build upon it for the future. To that end I offer this book.

Bright Blessings,

Cornwoman

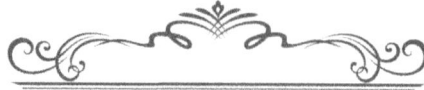

Introduction

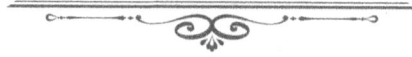

At the age of 14, I can remember sitting in a hot Southern Baptist church with my grandmother, watching an overweight preacher turn purple as he thundered on about Hell and damnation. In desperation, I looked out the window at beautiful blue hills and I thought that there was no love or spirituality in that church, only fear, guilt and self-righteousness. The true love and spirituality I so desperately sought was out there among the trees, close to the Earth.

I watched my grandmother sitting there, tears streaming down her face as she listened to the preacher, and I felt totally empty and separated from the process going on around me. I remember quite clearly then turning once again to the window and silently offering my life in service to the Earth Mother and the powers of the old ways.

It would be romantic to say at this point that, from then on, I never darkened a Christian church's door again, but that was not so. Being still a child with strong-minded relatives, I was limited in the liberties I could take. The spiritual commitment had been made, however, and from that point on, I intensified my studies with the elders whenever I could. I spent the rest of my teens in learning, and as an adult I wholeheartedly embraced the Native way, much to the disgust and fear of some of my relations.

The Native spiritual way was solely my path for more than thirty years. I learned a lot of invaluable knowledge from this tradition for which I will always be grateful, but the path I had so joyously embraced in my youth began to trouble and confine me by middle age. I began to question the Native tradition as now practiced, and the personal integrity of some medicine men teaching that tradition. Time and again I was hurt by the prejudice shown towards me as a Metis (half-breed) and I was disgusted by the Natives' non-acceptance of many whites who came to the reserve to learn, as well as by the whites' blind, uncritical acceptance of the unkind way they were treated.

I also found it hard to accept the sexual exploitation and other treatment many women received in this system, especially when they were on their Moon (menstruating). The women in traditional Native society are often excluded from ceremony for fear that their menstrual Blood would cause the ceremony to go awry. Such prejudice and fear left me feeling ashamed to be a woman, and fearful that in some way I might cause illness without even knowing it because of my Bleeding.

Unconsciously, at first, and later deliberately, I began to search for something beyond the confines of the tradition I grew up with and knew. In the early eighties my quest led me to the discovery of Wicca and the cult of the Goddess. It was like turning on a light in a dark room. For the first time I felt proud of my father's European heritage, because there were people in the Pagan tradition of Europe who honored and respected the Earth Mother as my Native Elders and I did.

Through the cult of the Goddess and knowledge of traditional European witchcraft, I began to feel like a whole human being. I learned a lot about self-worth and denial at this time in my life – lessons that had been missing from my training up till then. Embracing Wicca helped me to grow in ways that Native teachings never had.

For a while I was content with my new path, but as I learned more and attended more Pagan events, the old empty feeling returned, though for a different reason this time. My discontent now centered around the type of rituals I saw practiced by the New Age Pagan groups I met. I would leave so many gatherings feeling frustrated, like being in a state of arousal yet never reaching orgasm. I was frustrated because I knew from my Native training that there was a lot more to the practice of ritual than most Wiccans seemed to know.

Philosophically speaking, I liked what Wicca had to offer. Its respect for women on their Moon time was refreshing, making me feel good about myself, but traditional Native ceremony as practiced within Native communities was far more satisfying to me despite its difficulties. To go back to "the blanket," as it were, would mean putting up with a lot of unpleasant attitudes that I had hoped to leave behind me for good. But at least within the Native ceremonial system, I could find release if not fulfillment. What I needed was a ritual system that combined the best of both traditions.

When I tried to explain my ideas to other Pagans I knew, and suggested that we try some longer, more Indigenous, ritual forms at our gatherings, they usually looked at me blankly. Because they had never experienced anything similar to the way I had been taught, there was simply no common thread to unite us.

I finally realized that, like myself, most people who now claim to be Pagan chose that path as an adult. This meant that their Pagan religious training had no roots of any length. They had no elders to hand down teachings and experience (I do not consider anyone under sixty to be an elder) and no ritual tradition that is grounded in the land on which we live. When ungrounded people change their religion, usually it is only their beliefs that change, and not the ways in which they practice them. Unconsciously they fall back upon the old ritual form with which they are most familiar – in most cases, the Judeo-Christian one.

Let me illustrate. Imagine a typical modern Pagan rite. It begins, someone talks, we sing a short song, someone talks again, we talk more, sing, maybe dance a little, we end with a little talk and we all go home in an hour and a half. This example is over-simplified but essentially true. I saw the same basic format used by my Pagan friends and by the Baptist minister's service back home.

This is an uncomfortable analogy for most Pagans, who would like to think that they have left everything Christian behind. When I speak to them of Native rituals that last all night or go on for days at a time, they shake their heads or make a comment like "I couldn't possibly dance all night" because "I have to think of my health." Some of these same people are quite capable of partying all night, but for some reason they find an all-night ritual far more intimidating. I can understand their fear, because they don't know what is involved and whether they are capable of doing it, but nevertheless I find it intensely frustrating.

For a long time, I despaired of getting anywhere with the Pagan community, until I met Elizabeth Cogburn in the mid-1980's. Elizabeth taught a ceremonial style she called the Long Dance. This ceremony, to me, was a hybrid ritual combining elements from a variety of cultural sources. The ceremonies last several days and the participants preparation takes much longer. Her ceremonies combine, dance, drumming, and sacred theatre. For the first time, I saw a European tradition that had a potential for power and depth similar to what I was used to when attending Native events.

The structure used at a Long Dance is complex in many ways, yet it can be used by a number of different groups with different belief systems. Elizabeth is a learned Cabalist in the Hermetic tradition. When she performs the Long Dance, the teachings she offers with the dance come out of that tradition. I teach from a Native-Wiccan perspective, yet the form of the ceremonial that we share is similar. In spite of the different belief systems each teacher uses, a student from either group visiting the other would understand what was going on because the ritual structure is basically the same.

I have drawn heavily from Elizabeth's model for my own work, but my training in the Native way has given me a different perspective and slightly different approach to the ritual art from hers. I am grateful to her for providing me with a format from which I was able to develop a ceremonial system that combines the best of both my traditions.

The structure of ritual and the traditional teachings mentioned in these pages do not advocate any particular religion or belief system. The methods I employ can be adopted, with some modifications, by any group wishing to strengthen and deepen its ceremonial process, whether they are Pagan, Christian, or other.

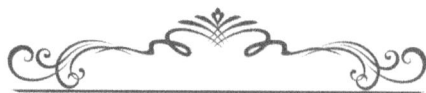

PART ONE

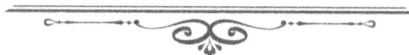

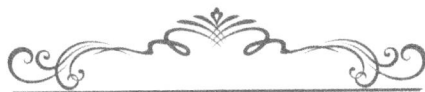

Chapter 1

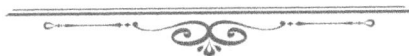

The Need for Ceremony –
Biological or Social?

After studying anthropology at university I came to the conclusion that one of the main things that distinguishes human kind from the rest of the warm-blooded creatures of this planet is our use of, and need for, religious ritual. The details of particular dig sites and carbon dating methods are all a blur after many years away from class, but what I do recall very vividly after all this time are the pictures of grave sites with bones laid out in the fetal position, covered with red ochre, with pottery and other tools laid nearby. Over the years I have often thought of those ancient ancestors. What prompted them to treat their dead in this manner? Were they told to do this by their Gods?

Modern scientists often speculate that it was "primitive man's" fear of his world that led to the development of religious practices. They cite the uncertainty of finding food, or unpredictable weather, as the reason for religious ritual to placate the Gods. I have always disagreed with that notion.

Based on my time living in the bush or among modern so-called "primitive" peoples, I know from personal experience that it is a deep sense of respect and love that motivates our lives, rather than one of cringing fear. If this is so for Indigenous People today, how much stronger must that deep sense of connection to the Earth have been for those Ancient Ones. Usually people only fear what they don't understand, and those growing up on the land learn to know it quite well at an early age.

Before the era when mass media bombardment began to stifle our psychic talents, our ability to connect and be in harmony with other life forms around us must have been very strong indeed. As a child and a young woman, I can remember hearing stories about Native elders who always knew exactly where to be to meet someone, on a certain day and in the right place, even though miles of bush with no radio or telephone separated them. Such abilities are far rarer than they once were, but they still exist as echoes of the power of the past. Such knowledge is based on a profound awareness of pulsating psychic energy fields that exist all around us.

The aim of these wise elders, from whatever racial or cultural group they may have come, was always to maintain a balance between these energy fields to create harmony in the world. Whenever humankind needed to affect these vibrational fields, they created some type of religious or "magical" ritual to achieve that end. That last statement is generally agreed upon by most authorities, but a less-asked question is whether that ritual response is biological in nature, or purely cultural in origin. Quite frankly I don't know, but I wonder.

Over the years the question has been put to me by different elders from a variety of different backgrounds. An old Scottish woman first brought it to my attention, claiming that certain racial stocks have more of the magical gift than others. Native elders that I know agree that the power can be passed through families; though that is not the only way it is passed. My teacher Elizabeth said it the best when she spoke of each person's biological need to experience the ecstatic communion with the divine. For Elizabeth, as for our ancestors, that need was fulfilled by practicing meaningful community ceremonials several times within the yearly cycle.

The possibility of having such a biological imperative coded into our very DNA is an interesting one – something to pleasantly debate with good friends around the fire on a long winter's night. I can't offer any scientific evidence to support such a claim, but I can say that deep down inside it feels right to me. I would also offer the argument that as I look around me, I see a deep hunger reflected in the faces of the people I meet, a craving for something more than can be found in the materialistic pleasures of our high-tech industrialized world.

Prior to our modern era, this inner fulfillment was offered by religious rites. The Catholics had the feasts of the saints, the Pagans of Europe had their cross-quarter days, and Native Americans had events like the Navajo Beauty Way ceremony and the Winter Dances of the Northwest. All cultures had, and some still do have, these highly-evolved ritual traditions to honor the divine and keep the balance of natural forces in order.

Though the religious rituals of the industrialized West are but weak shadows of their former selves, I would argue that the biological drive is still within us, insisting that it be acknowledged. I believe this drive still exists within each of us, though its fulfillment isn't usually beneficial. Taken out of the realm of the sacred where its power could be channeled into creativity and healing, it is now secularized into gang rituals, alcohol and drug use, and rock concerts.

All of these activities are either destructive or chaotic, a sad mockery of the balanced healing rituals of sacred life. Our world stands at the brink of destruction because so many have forgotten how to fulfill this bio-cultural need in a healthy, balanced way.

As caring human beings, we must come together to form functioning communities that can live in harmony with each other and the Earth. There is a lot of talk about just that today, but what is missing from this talk, and, in general, from the communal experiments to date, is a dynamic ceremonial structure to bring and keep the community together. I would offer, as a living example of a workable community model for those interested in forming communities, the Pueblo Indians of the Southwestern United States.

An anthropologist once claimed that these people spend two-thirds of their lives either preparing for, or performing, religious ceremonies. No wonder they are called the Peaceful People. With so much time devoted to the sacred, there is little left over to make war.

In their system, conflicts are handled in ritualized ways, thus avoiding violence so that group harmony is maintained. The tragedy of our modern society is that too few people have lived the spiritual community process, and so don't know practical ways to re-create it for themselves in the larger society. The root of the word "community" is the word "common." Along with economics and politics, religious rituals need to be shared by those wishing to live together. For many of us, there is a desire not to blindly parrot the decaying forms of the modern world.

We must create a new community and ceremonial system, unfortunately for most of us there are few signposts or guidelines out there, and often it may seem like making your way through heavy mud, one step forward and two steps back. In the last thirty years there have been many attempts at community-building, and almost all have failed, leaving their members frustrated and disillusioned, wondering why it didn't work. Once again, as world conditions worsen, there is a new urgency to re-establish working community models that can act as a guide for the growth of future generations.

Some have chosen to look for these guidelines in the teachings of ancient religions from various parts of the world. The Far East, Wicca, and Native Americans all have much to offer, but we need to take care when we remove their ancient wisdom from its cultural context and apply it piecemeal to our modern society. Too often teachings are parroted without knowledge of their deeper meaning. To strengthen your understanding of whatever ancient system you choose, I suggest that you must also be willing to take on the ceremonial patterns and instructional methods of these ancient traditions.

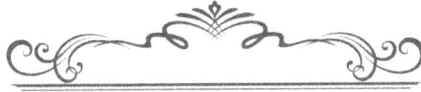

Chapter 2

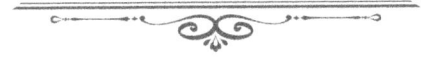

Traditional Apprenticeship
Versus Modern Teaching Methods

I consider ritual to be an art. Like any other art form, to be really good at it takes knowledge, talent, experience, and commitment. In practical terms, this means years of hard work and study. Unfortunately, this idea is often hard to get across to students growing up in an era where quick fixes and fast food meals are a way of life.

Modern society is based on the impersonality of the assembly line and mass production. The concept of craftsmanship in any area of human endeavor has almost disappeared from our lives. I believe it is an important concept, however, and that we must re-introduce craftsmanship to our work as practicing ceremonialists if we want to achieve similar results to those our ancestors accomplished.

Throughout most of our long history, young people learned a trade (including that of a Indigenous spiritual doctor) through a slow process called an apprenticeship. At an early age, a child would be sent to live with an elder, or a master of his or her craft. During this time, the apprentice would be expected to do a lot of hard work and chores for the elder that had little or nothing to do with his or her training in the craft itself. This work was seen as a service and mark of respect to the elder, and it also helped to pay for the apprentice's lessons. As the master observed the student over time, he or she would gradually be given more work and responsibility within the craft by the master. This system gave each of them time to learn about the other.

At first the apprentice learned through observation and memorization. The young were expected to copy the elder's technique and not ask many questions. "You do it this way because we have always done it this way." In time, practice would start to bring understanding, and eventual explanations would be tempered by the apprentice's own insights and experience.

Some of the more lenient craft masters may have been willing to answer questions, even from a very junior apprentice. However, the training was still almost entirely practical rather than theoretical, and certainly apprentices have always done whatever menial labor their masters required.

In a somewhat modified form, this is how most indigenous apprentices learn their craft today. The same is true in families with an inherited tradition of Wicca. Nowadays, the apprentice does not always live with the elder, but is expected to live near enough to be at the service of the old one whenever a ceremony or healing needs to be performed. In the modern world, this type of training will mean years of sacrifice for the student; it may mean that it will be hard to hold down a regular job and support a family and still do the ceremonial "work" required.

In the past, the apprentice being trained by the Elder would have been taken care of by the community while he or she was undergoing the training, as an investment in the future health of the members of the community. This is still done, to a point, in some places, but because of the breakdown in community life in most areas the student is forced to be more self-reliant than previously.

Structure and authority are important parts of this traditional system, needed to maintain a high quality of practice. In many modern professions, such as medicine and law, standards are maintained by the fact that authority is legally needed to practice these professions, and these standards are enforced by those already having the authority and by the legal system itself. (Because of the actions of the AMA and other organizations, for instance, practicing medicine without a license is a criminal offense in many jurisdictions.)

Within their own communities, Indigenous healers and spiritual leaders are seen as being as much of a professional as are doctors or ministers within white society. For this reason, standards do exist for practicing the ceremonial arts, and those standards are maintained, not by a formal organization like the AMA, but by the apprenticeship system and by a loosely-knit council of Spiritual Elders. In the traditional Native system, an apprentice would not be allowed to do a ritual until and unless he or she was given the authority by an Elder to do so.

Because of past abuses by doctors, lawyers, politicians, and other authority figures, as well as by cult figures who deliberately encourage their followers to give over their free will to the cult leaders, modern people are all too well aware of the potential dangers of granting authority to new or unfamiliar kinds of spiritual practitioners. Abuses of power (power of males over females, power of parents over children, power of church elders and ministers over their congregations) are so pervasive in our society that they have led those seeking to create new community patterns to a sometimes unreasonable fear of exploitation and to rebellion against authority in any form.

It is important to establish boundaries, to take care of oneself, and to prevent oneself from being exploited, but sometimes it is wise to rely on the guidance of an experienced person, who can warn the novice of dangers and pitfalls that he could not otherwise avoid.

Many people who have now chosen to follow a Pagan path grew up not taking their parents' religion (if any) very seriously, and so, unconsciously, perhaps, they tend to view their Pagan practices lightly. Most Pagans have an attitude that anyone can do a ritual, because they have never experienced the kind of ritual that not everyone can perform. They have a lingering doubt and a feeling that they may be just playing a game anyway, so what difference does it make who leads a ritual? Thus, they are unaware of the potential dangers involved in tampering, even superficially, with the magic arts.

Some of the dangers that modern Pagans may be unaware of (or disregard) include the boomerang effect, the possibility of psychic attack, the effects of leaving oneself ungrounded after a ritual, and the unwanted effects that may occur if the intent of a ceremony is either harmful or unclear. (These pitfalls will be explained in detail later in this book.)

Apprenticeship is a powerful method of learning, and it is usually a safe method because of its reliance on structure and authority in practicing a trade. But it is also slow by modern standards.

Problems arise when people living in modern urban areas come to traditional teachers wanting to learn their craft. I include here both Native and non-Native students, because both have grown up in a system where their only exposure to learning has come through the public schools, and so they have only a very vague idea about traditional teaching methods.

How many times have I heard some young disillusioned person say, "Oh, I went to study with so-and-so and it was nothing but a waste of my time. I didn't learn a thing. I was there three months and all I did was clean her house or chop his wood or babysit their kids."

Such young people do not understand the concept of apprenticeship and traditional teaching methods. They were unable to learn what was there to be learnt because the lessons were not laid out in a manner they were used to. There were no school books, no homework assignments, no lectures or trips to the library. In such cases, everybody suffers; the elders despair of passing on their knowledge and skills, and the young are confused by the old teaching method, and return to the city bitter at the old ways for not meeting their needs for instant results.

Some traditional elders are adapting and allowing their materials to be written down in books to prevent their knowledge from disappearing completely. But there is a lot of controversy about this within all traditional communities, be they Native North American, Australian, European Asian or African. I personally see advantages and disadvantages in both systems, so perhaps the answer lies in a balance between the two forms of teaching.

The old apprenticeship method, be it for Indigenous healer or smith-crafter, is slow but thorough. This system gives the personality time to mature before taking on certain responsibilities. (Some people may choose to train for a craft later in life, after they are already mature. Since these older students have already had considerable life experience to temper their judgements, they may need less time to achieve similar results, thus a shorter apprenticeship. Nevertheless, at least for the profession of spiritual healer, these older pupils still need to go through all the same steps of their training; they may simply be able to progress through some of them faster.)

One disadvantage of the apprenticeship system is that our modern communities, even Indigenous ones, are not very cohesive anymore, and there is little local or national support available for the budding spiritual healer as there once would have been. Taking a nine-to-five job in the "real world" is often a necessity, but must mean less time available for the spiritual training. Another disadvantage is that an apprentice can only learn what the master can teach, so all the master's personal biases and limitations will be reflected in his or her apprentices.

There are three types of teaching styles that I am aware of. Some teachers are so wise that people learn just by being around them. I would call these the "gentle teachers", who teach by unconditional love and the example of their lives. The second kind is the strict disciplinarian, who teaches with a very structured system, where the students have specific tasks they have to do, and discipline is very important. The third type of teacher is the trickster, and they're hard to describe. They mostly teach through shock, and they do things to startle and upset their pupils. A good example of the trickster teacher is Don Juan in Carlos Castaneda's books. Apprentices may need different teaching styles at different times in their lives, or they may deliberately choose certain teachers in order to learn certain lessons.

Modern teaching methods have their advantages too, just as apprenticeships do. In schools, students receive a lot of facts and information very quickly. While mastering this bewildering array of information, a student gets feedback on his or her abilities at regular intervals as test scores are posted. There are also advantages to learning from several teachers and not just one, because the student gains a broader perspective and is less likely to pick up biases from a single teacher. With this method, a student can attend school part-time and still have a paying job.

Because the educational materials are mass-produced, there is little room for individuality, and students on either end of the learning spectrum can be frustrated by material that is either too difficult or too easy. Perhaps the primary disadvantage of the modern system, however, is that people graduate with a lot of facts that they have learned from books, but they have no practical experience to balance them out—they have no idea of how to use the facts they have learned. The key question here is whether the student really is learning or is just memorizing facts.

To give a spiritual example: using modern teaching techniques, New Age teachers can teach previously untrained people how to do such ancient mystery arts as fire-walking within an afternoon. The question here, however, is what have you really learned by performing this feat in one afternoon? In ancient mystery schools and other Indigenous traditions, such a technique as fire-walking would have taken the student years to prepare for. Only the wise old elders would possess such power. All the years of preparation meant that when the walk finally came, it was a life-transforming event whose power lasted throughout the rest of the student's life.

With only the time investment of an afternoon, it is often easy to slip back into the old destructive patterns of thinking in spite of the power felt during the walk itself. Spiritual teachers who use this technique have told me about their frustration at seeing their students slip back into old habits even though they know better.

Traditional elders would claim that knowledge gained too quickly cannot be retained. (Do you remember cramming for exams in high school? How much of what you studied did you remember a week later?) From my own personal experience I would tend to agree with the Elders.

One of the truly great wonders of the New Age is this ability to take these ancient mysteries out of the realm of religious dogma and prove that they can be performed by common people. Such knowledge can give us the power and confidence to shape our own futures, but it needs to be balanced with some of the tools of the past. In this, I refer to the use of ceremony.

Prolonging the preparation, and creating an elaborate ritual to honor and celebrate a gift of power such as a fire-walk, will increase the transformative effects of the event. This is a brief example of how the old and new teaching methods can be reconciled to meet the needs of our modern world.

Before leaving the topic of apprenticeship, I want to discuss another point that has a bearing on this topic, and that is the concern of time. Traditional teaching methods take time, lots of time. Not only are there a vast number of people who would like to learn but have trouble adding another commitment to their days, but there are also a growing number who feel we, as a race, have little time left before the world is destroyed by nuclear war, environmental disaster, economic collapse, or other world-shaking catastrophes.

Almost all of the world's religions have prophecies that predict the world's end. Many people strongly believe (or fear) that that time is coming soon. This often leads to a desperate need to learn the old ways as a means of personally coping with those fears. Traditional ceremonial systems have a lot to offer, but not, alas, at the expense of cutting corners. By their very nature, they take time to learn and perfect, and there is no way around that.

This issue will come up again when we discuss community building, but let me just say that, in my opinion, some compromises, in a limited way, can be made to shorten the time taken, but the student must approach the learning process, not with an air of desperation, but with the confidence that he or she will learn what is needed in the time allotted for him or her on this planet. Any other approach will only be counterproductive in the end.

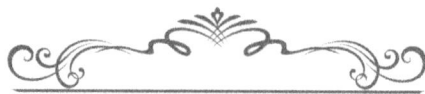

Chapter 3

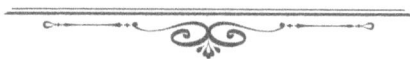

Energy Exchange and Respect

The issue of respect for, and service to, an elder is a subject not well understood today. In practical terms it may mean being someone's "go-fer," as one disgusted young woman claimed she was not about to be. But to be or not to be a go-fer is not the question. It is more a matter of honoring the sacred power that is working through a particular teacher rather than of honoring the person.

Somewhere back in the European past, people took a wrong turning, confusing the divine in a person with the person himself. Because of this, there is a whole segment of history where half-mad kings and emperors forgot that they were there to spiritually serve the people. They ruled their domains and claimed their offices as a personal right of inheritance or of wealth and power, and enforced that right with strength of arms. Modern politicians, and even more so the military-industrial complex (which controls much of modern politics even in democracies), rule with almost as much absolute power as divinely-maintained kings.

This has led to a deep mistrust of authority of any kind that is very wide-spread among those of the New Age seeking to create a new world reality. In some sense, I would argue that this rebellion has gone too far the other way, almost to the extreme of throwing the baby out with the bath-water.

This failure to accept authority has led in time, for many people, to the point of directionless drifting. One can learn a lot from exploring the inner self, but at some point it is our nature as humans to need guidance from those wiser than ourselves. To do this, we need to accept, even in a limited way, the divine power manifested in another person to guide and protect one's self. Doing service to an elder teacher as part of the apprenticeship program shows respect, and should in no way be seen as demeaning to the person performing the tasks.

There is a basic law of the universe working here that must be satisfied in some way. That is to say that in all exchanges of goods, or in this case information of a spiritual nature, there must be an energy exchange on the part of both persons for the universe to be balanced. The teacher pays by passing on the information he or she knows how to teach. The student may pay as well, by a gift of money, other goods, or service. The student won't get the benefit of the teaching (at least not the full benefit) if it is not paid for in some way.

Material goods or service must be willingly given, a sacrifice of the self to the sacred. It is not easy, but there is a great gift to the self in learning that truth. Sometimes the service may seem like being a "go fer," though if the student treats the service in that manner, she will miss the point and not get much out of the experience.

The other thing that confuses the issue is people's views around money. There is an unwritten law in the West that a workshop can only be good if it costs a lot. Many people trying to live and teach in a traditional style do not like to charge money because that is not how they were taught. In return for their teachings, though, they do expect some recompense.

For example, if you plan to attend a sweat lodge ceremony, there may not be a charge, but the people putting on the sweat had to put out time and money to prepare the site, get the wood, and countless other chores. When people arrive for the sweat then leave without offering anything in exchange, either more wood, cleaning up, or even money, it creates an energy imbalance that will lead to frustration and hard feelings. Elders expect people to know these things without being told, and often their own personal codes of not asking for payment will prevent them from mentioning it.

The old traditions have broken down in so many places that what we need today is a mediator—someone to instruct the student in his or her role without the elder needing to do so. Most of the time such lapses are not done out of disrespect or a desire to free-load. They are more likely done out of ignorance of a system of learning that has almost been forgotten in our modern urban world. It is, however, something that the modern student wishing to be instructed in the older traditions needs to be sensitive to.

In a similar vein, there is the whole issue of that filthy green stuff, "money." As a ceremonial facilitator, I constantly ponder this question. Should I charge? How much should I charge? If I charge a high enough price that people will think my event is worth attending, then I will limit my students to a class of people who can financially afford to come, yet may not be serious or committed to the work. If, on the other hand, I don't charge at all (or very little), I may not cover expenses, or have enough to pay my bills and live, so I can continue to do the work I've been guided to do.

These are very deep philosophical issues that most teachers of good conscience struggle with. I have decided that what works for me, to have peace with myself, is to offer my teachings to whoever asks on a donation basis. I leave it totally up to the students to give what they feel my help has been worth. It isn't easy, but I try to have trust in the powers that I serve that I will be taken care of, and just leave it at that, and usually that is enough.

Sometimes it backfires and I am taken advantage of materially, however. I recall a class of ten to twelve people who put in, week after week, less than ten dollars all told, while my expenses were twenty-five to thirty dollars. Physically I lost, but I figure on a spiritual level they lost even more for trying to take advantage, because they all had good corporate or government jobs and could afford more than what they chose to give.

I felt unable to discuss my needs with them, but if I had had a mediator, that person could have talked to my students in my absence, and explained to them about respect for their teacher and about the need for an energy exchange.

An important point is that both in the modern and the traditional teaching systems, there is some form of payment by the student for the teachings. In the modern system, the teacher asks for money; in the traditional system, the student offers service. When a modern student tries to study under a traditional teacher, each one expects the other to arrange the payment. If no payment is therefore arranged, the teacher feels cheated (thinking the student is unwilling to pay), and the student either believes that he has gotten away with something, or feels that the teaching must be worthless since no payment was demanded.

What happens when a traditional student tries to learn from a modern teacher? Schools will generally insist on money as payment, as may the more mercenary individual teachers. Other teachers may accept service in lieu of money, but the teacher may feel he is doing a favor by waiving his usual fee, and the student may feel like a charity case, inferior to other students who are really paying. Some modern teachers may also exploit the student by demanding more service than the equivalent in money, because service is seen as inferior to money.

Thus, respect for the teacher and some form of energy exchange are necessary, and the form of the exchange must be discussed and clarified beforehand to prevent misunderstandings and a breakdown in communication between teacher and student. People wishing to build a new community and ceremonial system must be sure to handle these issues in some deliberate way, rather than assuming they will take care of themselves.

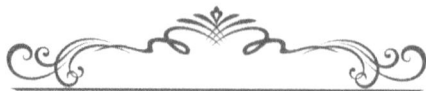

Chapter 4

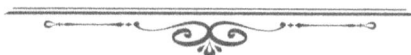

Motivation and Ethics

Any student who has chosen a particular spiritual path needs to ask him or herself what the reasons are for choosing that path. The elders say that a person's motivations are what makes the difference between walking a spiritual path and one of sorcery or black magic. Both paths to power must answer to the same natural laws and often use the same ritual tools and ceremonies. It is the human agent's purpose that makes the difference.

Upon quick reflection, it might appear that it would be easy to determine what is good or bad in one's work, but upon deeper consideration, these areas may be a little grayer than at first appears. To illustrate, let me cite two examples – are they spiritual or sorcery?

Example one: A group of friends have gathered together to do a healing ceremony for another friend who is not present, but has just learned that she has cancer. During the ceremony, they imagine her standing in the centre of their circle and they pour healing energy into her image.

Example two: A fundamentalist preacher stands before his congregation in the height of prayer. Everyone is very emotionally charged. The preacher asks his church to join with him in calling down the wrath of God upon a sinner who has violated God's holy commandments.

Spirituality or sorcery? I would argue that both groups are guilty of practicing, if not black, then very dirty gray magical arts. The first group, the healing circle, mean nothing but good, but they do not have the cancer patient's permission to try to heal her. No matter how noble the motives may be, when you try to rescue someone who has not asked for your help, then you are robbing that person of his or her free will. Some people need their disease process in order to grow spiritually. In trying to help, you could be setting back their growth by a whole lifetime. In the specific case given, for instance, the

24

woman may need to accept the fact that she is not immortal, that sooner or later she will die, before she tries to heal herself. Failure to accept her own mortality will maintain her permanently in the state of denial that all of us are prone to as children.

The old people say that you must never help someone unless they ask for it and are willing to do some type of energy exchange to show their commitment to the whole process. It would be permissible for the healing circle to ask whether she wants their magical support, but they must not proceed without her consent. Sometimes the issue is evaded by psychically asking permission for a healing to be done. Unless one in the circle is so much in tune with the woman as to be certain of being in true telepathic contact with her, they should ask for and receive her consent verbally and not just mentally – it is too easy to let wishful thinking delude one into believing one has received an answer.

The people in the second example are equally guilty of sorcery, because even though they sit in a church and call on the name of the Christian God, they are using the energy built up during the service to curse rather than to bless. Despite the appearance of God's just punishment on the sinner, it is still a curse. Whether the sinner actually committed the sin, and just how dreadful a sin it was, makes no difference to the fact that the congregation has cursed him. Though rarely thought of in this way by Christians, this holy cursing is a kind of sorcery.

Both religion and magic are subject to the same laws, though we tend to forget that. There is a natural law of the universe called, in Wicca, the "three-fold law." This law, in essence, states that whatever you think, say, or do comes back to you three times over. It is interesting to me that much of the time, when Christians feel that they are under attack by the devil, what they are really experiencing are the effects of the three-fold law. The number "three" is not necessarily exact; some acts seem to come back to us much more than three-fold. The point is that they come back multiplied. This applies to acts of kindness as well as to acts of revenge.

Many modern texts and teachers of Wicca are very lax in their ethical teachings. Most of them mention ethics, but some pay it no more than lip-service. Some books even offer spells for blasting undesirables such as rapists and mass murderers. No matter how justified a person may feel, a curse is a curse, and if you perform it, be prepared to face the effects of the three-fold law.

That is a fact that can't be denied, even though sorcerers throughout the ages have tried to deny it.

Ritual is a tool. It is neither good nor bad in itself. Human will and emotion determine its direction. When you curse or blast another, you are working from a place of fear and revenge, and that is always a dangerous place from which to do ritual. Coming from a place of love is always your best bet, and if you can't be clear that your underlying motivations are beneficial to all, then try to solve your problem in some more conventional way. Some Wiccans believe that, while it is not permissible (or safe) to curse someone, it is permissible to do an "instant karma" spell on them. When in my youth I tried to do an instant karma spell, what I found was that, not only did the person I cast the spell on get his deserved karma, but I got my instant karma too, and I didn't like it. So if you're planning to do this kind of spell-casting, make sure there's nothing in your past you want to catch up with you!

But what motivates people to choose a ceremonial path as opposed to a more conventional religious philosophy? The answer to that is quite complicated. What I have observed is that in different groups there are different reasons behind people's choices. In the modern Pagan groups, three types of reasons often prevail. The first group chooses ritual and the shamanic arts as another tool to add to more traditional methods of psychotherapy. The aim of these people is self-growth and the healing of old traumas. Examples would be women's support groups and healing circles that heal old traumas by the use of ritual.

Another type of person chooses to do ritual or spell-casting to solve his or her personal problems in order to avoid looking at them. An example is a woman who does a spell to get rid of an abusive partner – her third abusive partner, yet she is unwilling to look at the underlying reasons why she constantly chooses this type of person.

The third type sees mastering a spiritual path as a way to make money. To these individuals, their time investment must be paid for by their future students or patients. I can become very angry with this last group because, in most cases, the indigenous elders they learned from did not charge them thousands of dollars for their knowledge. To turn around and charge big bucks for what was freely and trustingly given smacks too strongly of a new type of imperialistic exploitation for me. Not to get off on a personal tangent, the point is that in all three categories, the needs of the person are placed first, not the needs of the community or the society.

In other cultures, any of the above reasons may be present in a given individual, but they are not seen as the main reason to choose a religious path, as is too often the case in Western society. The old people say that a good spirit-doctor (shaman) does not choose his calling, he/she is chosen by the spirits when there is a need for him/her in their community. When a spirit-doctor is given the power to heal, that one becomes a servant of the power that flows through them. If someone is ill and requests healing, then the spirit-doctor is obliged to do what they can, regardless of what his/her personal preference in the matter may be. If he/she doesn't respect that obligation to serve and use his/her healing power, it will leave that person and find another channel.

This type of calling is not for ego trippers. It is hard, self-sacrificing service to "the people." I do not mean to imply that only among Natives can you find this type of dedication to the service of humanity; far from it. Such people are present in every culture. I am merely stating the examples with which I am familiar. And perhaps the modern world has to re-examine its idea of healing and service to the community.

An example from Western society of a few years ago is the "old country doctor," who had (at his best) the same ideal of service without thought of himself. Many people deplore his loss, contrasting it to modern doctors – always on the golf course, charging huge fees, no house calls, refusing to treat the poor, etc. Probably few old doctors were as good, and few new doctors are as bad, as these stereotypes would have them, of course. Nevertheless, the old ideal of service to the community was similar to the Native ideal of the herbal and spirit-doctor, and is one that the would-be spiritual healers of today would do well to imitate.

Commitment to a spiritual calling has high costs, both to yourself and to your family. The spirit doctor must make it a life's work, and must go where they are asked and do what is needed. If he or she is good, that person may rarely have a day off. However, there are also benefits to this path. Among other things, there is a great satisfaction in helping others and knowing that you make a difference. In addition, there is a intoxicating high in feeling the power run through you, but remember that this high can become addictive, and the true spiritual healer must beware of ego-tripping.

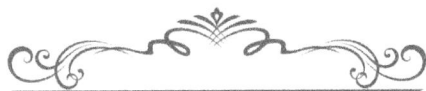

Chapter 5

The Evolution of a Ritual Group

The purpose of most traditional rites in aboriginal societies is to bring harmony and unity to the village. To do this consistently, a rigid structural system must be devised. New Age Pagan rites are alive with creativity and experimentation, but contain little structure and are thus very fluid. No rules, no structure – their essence is, "to go with the flow."

The advantage of the "go with the flow" ritual seems to be that the participants can gain a lot of self-awareness and experience in a short time, because there is no authoritarian structure to inhibit their growth. The disadvantage of this type of practice lies in its inconsistency. These rites can be absolutely beautiful or totally disastrous, depending on where they are held, who shows up, how they feel that day, and so on.

Most modern Pagans treat this phenomenon as a perfectly normal state of affairs, but in most other parts of the world that still practice older traditions, such inconsistency would be treated as a major failure of the rite. Cultures that lay out a blueprint of their ritual practices and follow it strictly have much more consistent results; they need to, because, as they see it, these cultures rely on their ceremonies to keep the world in balance. They are not as concerned with "personal growth" as they are with the welfare of the world as a whole.

In my experience, "do as you feel" ritual seems to be a stage that most groups go through as they develop, rather than being an end in itself. What I have observed is that most New Age groups (especially women's groups) begin with a "do as you feel" format, which is intended to break down old patterns of patriarchal authority, but if they stay together long enough, they eventually adopt a more structured format, perhaps with a rotating system of leadership and authority.

The model chosen may be one of changing structure and leadership, but structure will be there, and rightly so, because to live on the physical plane is to be governed by natural laws. To live without rules is to live in chaos, and that is to be out of balance with life. Women, in particular, often resist becoming leaders (of ritual or anything else). This is partly from a lack of self-confidence and partly from a reluctance to re-create anything resembling a patriarchal authority structure. However, those groups that don't choose some kind of structure usually stagnate and die from lack of committed direction and leadership.

I would suggest to anyone wishing to form or join a ritual group that they do some study about group process. There are different stages of development that all groups pass through as they evolve. Many groups are formed, but once the honeymoon is over and conflicts arise, the group begins to disband. It might be comforting to know that conflict is a stage that groups all go through, and that it will pass. Once past, the members who have stuck it out will really get down to serious learning and working together. The process will also empower their rituals, because at that point the group will start to function as a group, not just as an assortment of individuals.

Most people join a group with only a vague idea of what they want out of the experience and what they are willing to give to the group in return. One of the best ways to avoid conflicts and power plays is to get clear as soon as possible what it is that the participants want as a group. To do effective ritual, the group must become a working unit that has a life of its own beyond the sum of its individual members. This is a lot easier when members have a vision in common.

It is also important to know that a group that meets regularly to perform ritual together may or may not wish to take on the duties of a therapy group or a study group. That all needs to be decided as they meet, because one group (unless it is very intimate) may not be able to meet all its members' needs. Like romantic relationships, we need outside interests to bring life into the "marriage." Unless the group chooses to do therapy along with its magical work, a member having old traumas re-awakened by a ceremony may need to seek a support group focusing on those traumas, rather than monopolize group time and energy for that purpose. This is true especially for large group events at major holidays.

Lastly, bear in mind that ritual groups, or groups in general, have a life span, just like people. They are born, they grow and change, and they die. Sometimes we cling on to a very dysfunctional group when it should be allowed to die a natural death so that it can be born anew at a later time, perhaps in a different context or with different members.

‹❦›

RITUAL AS LIVING BEING

When I teach and perform ceremonies, I proceed from the assumption that, once the ritual process has begun, the ceremony takes on a life of its own. The ritual, in a sense, becomes a living being with a destiny and needs of its own, beyond those of the human beings participating in its pattern. My teacher Elizabeth Cogburn used to say, "You do not choose to Long Dance; the Dance chooses you." In my experience, this is true. The dancers become like different cells in a ritual body. Like heart, brain, or liver, they have their place and function within the whole process. This concept does not mean that there is no spontaneity or freedom of individual expression; it merely means that they happen within boundaries. In short, the needs of the ritual come before those of the individual and his or her ego.

The performance of large group seasonal rites is not the time or the place for displays of emotional distress or for rescue work. A small group setting, focused around the cycles of the Moon, is better suited to this type of inner work. In that setting, if members choose to, they can establish trust and support for one another. This long-term intimacy permits deep sharing.

Seasonal rites, especially those dedicated to another purpose, have neither the time nor the energy needed to work on deep personal issues. These rites are best used for celebration and to summon the seasonal Sacred Powers. In a seasonal ritual lasting over a number of days, where trust and support have time to develop, some therapy and trance work could, and should, be done; but by the whole group, not just for one individual's benefit. To treat one person's traumas in depth requires a special ceremony (if indeed ceremony is the chosen treatment), not just an add-on to a ritual with another intent.

It is a natural tendency for the unbalanced and inexperienced person to respond emotionally to the energies raised during a ceremony, but it does present a problem when participants disrupt a ritual to satisfy their own needs. People who disrupt a ritual may or may not be ego-tripping. Their motivation is often unclear, even to them. Usually it rises out of deep hurt and need for attention and support that they don't know how to get in other ways. As participants in a ritual, however, they have a responsibility to the ceremony and the other participants. They need to be willing to give to as well as take from the energy field.

The idea of subordinating the demands of the ego to the needs of the group's balance and harmony is not a well-understood concept among modern Pagans. But this is an important concept to understand, if new and existing spiritual communities are to develop and grow in these times. In aboriginal societies, people learn early the value of sharing and the concept of self-sacrifice for "the people."

One of the oldest prayers that I know translates as, "Oh, great mystery, give me strength that my people may live." This is a very simple yet profound prayer, stating quite clearly the meaning behind much of the traditional Native teachings. If I could think of a prayer that reflects modern society in general, it might be, "Oh, God, give me strength so that I may live and acquire more material goods." From this point of view, the New Age has come a long way; their prayer might be, "Oh, God or Goddess, give me strength to discover more about myself and grow spiritually."

The point that I am trying to make here is that, in both these non-aboriginal examples, the centre of the prayer, like the focus of many rituals performed today, is the individual and not the group well-being. This is an over-simplification that many will take issue with, and I would agree that it is a generalization, but even in such altruistic causes as the environmental movement, people often find it hard to set their egos aside and work for the common good.

Since the 1800's, humankind has made a lot of discoveries in the realm of individual freedoms, but if we want to survive on this planet much longer, we must take these lessons and learn once again how to function in a group mind with an evolved individual consciousness within it. Responding to ritual as if it were a living being in itself is one step towards a group mind.

This means asking yourself what you have to offer the ceremony, as well as asking what you hope to get from the experience. Many people fear this process, believing that they will become like zombies with no will of their own. That is possible, but it is an extreme. Individual self-growth as a life-time obsession is equally extreme, and it is destructive to both the person and the community. What is needed is a balance in all things between the needs of the individual and the group. Structured ritual can act as a bond, bringing people together and demonstrating how the needs of group and individual can mesh.

Among the Pueblo Indians, different groups in the community are responsible for different seasonal rituals. They divide up the work for practical as well as spiritual reasons. Preparations for their rites often take months and no one person or group could possibly be responsible for every ceremony within the year.

On an island where I once lived, there are several small pagan groups which meet separately at the new or full Moons. Representatives from these groups get together to plan larger island-wide seasonal rituals. Different people plan different rituals; thus, no one person or group takes on so much work as to suffer burnout. This system works well, but in my opinion it could be improved still further by spending more time in planning and preparing for these rites, and by lengthening the events themselves.

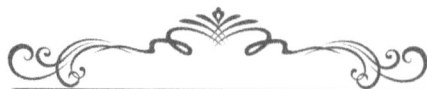

Chapter 6

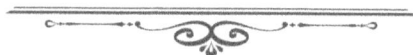

Symbols, Patterns, and the Ritual Process

When I use the word "symbol" I am referring to a physical object, a word, or a mental image that represents a broader and usually more abstract idea. Webster's Dictionary defines "symbol," in part, as "a visible sign of something invisible." Symbols can be used as a sort of spiritual short-hand. Let me illustrate. If I use a blue cloth on my altar to represent the element of water, I am using a symbol, because cloth, no matter what its colour, will never be the same as real water.

If every time I catch myself growing angry for no apparent reason, I imagine myself taking off a horrible mask so that I can see what lies beneath the anger, then that is a different type of symbol. In that case, the mask represents my emotional block and my unwillingness to seek out the deeper source of my feelings.

Language itself is nothing more than a system of symbols. All ceremonies rely quite heavily on the use of systems of symbols to represent ideas and beliefs that in turn give the world shape and significance. In short, our symbols determine how we perceive and react to the world around us. Many a war has been fought over which side has the "true" set of symbols by which to live.

The point, to me, is not which person or group has the "true" system of symbols, but that we all have a system and that they all work, for the people who created them and use them. Granted, some symbols, and some systems of symbols, are more balanced and life-affirming than others. Ethical issues aside, all systems do what they need to do to help the people who live by them to create and define their reality.

For those of us who practice the ceremonial arts, this is a freeing concept, because when doing any magic or ritual, our aim should be to restructure and redefine reality. To do that we need to redefine the system of symbols we use, or create a new one that will help us reshape our reality to include new possibilities.

Most of us cannot conceive how much power we actually have to define our reality. In school, scientists teach us that this world is a solid concrete fact with certain unbreakable laws. For example, fire will always burn you. If this is true, then what makes it possible for a person to walk across hot coals without being burned?

The Fire-Walk is not trickery or illusion, I can swear to that; I have walked a bed of hot coals about fifteen feet long twice so far in my life, with no burns at all on my feet. Scientists have given certain rationalizations of how they believe the act is accomplished, but what seems to me to happen is that the fire-walker merely changes his or her symbol system of reality to include the fact that fire will not burn under certain conditions.

On your own, you probably would not have enough personal power to overcome your old pattern of thinking that says that if you are stupid enough to walk on those coals, you are going to barbeque your feet. But in a setting where the other group members can support you in your new belief, the chances are very good that you will walk and not be burned. This does not mean that the next time you touch a hot pot in the kitchen you won't get a blister. It usually only means that under certain conditions your programming for reality has slipped enough to allow an alternative view of the world to exist alongside the old view.

Fire walking raises some interesting issues about how we could change our reality if only we tried. It is possible that the usual view, i.e. that fire will burn you, is the automatic one that the physical world follows unless we interfere. I mean that fire burning us is not so just because our culture believes it, but because it is the default way the world works. (After all, animals get burned too.)

If this is so, then fire-walking is possible only in an altered state of consciousness, and a hot pot will burn even an experienced fire-walker because he has not had time to enter the altered state. Also, it takes power to enter and remain in that state, so how long you can stay there depends on your personal power and your experience in such matters.

Let me offer another more common example from my past experience. Years ago, I learned how to set up and use something called a medicine wheel. Medicine wheels have four different-colored sticks, cloths, or altars to represent the four cardinal points on the compass. The purpose of the sticks (or whatever) is to define sacred space and to act as protection for the people inside the wheel. This description is over-simplified, but my point here is not a discourse on the wheel.

When I began to travel and saw how other peoples use the medicine wheel, I saw that, though every culture seemed to have one, they were all using different colors to represent the four directions. This confused and worried me. How could all these different systems work, and which of them was the true system? What was the real way to set up and use a medicine wheel? Was the one that I was using right, or was it one of the wrong ways? I think that most of us have asked similar questions of ourselves and our beliefs at some time or other.

I finally came to the conclusion that it did not matter what colors I used, or what system I used to set it up; all were equally valid. What mattered was the pattern as a whole, not its pieces. So if I was working within a Native pattern that called for a medicine wheel, I had better use one, or the ritual would be incomplete. But if I was using another system that did not call for a medicine wheel, then I needn't bother. A particular set of directional colors was of significance only within a given cultural context; they had no real influence on the working other than that.

When I was doing Tarot readings, I discovered that it was possible to create my own system and have it work as well as older, more established card layouts. As I became more experienced with the cards, I found that the traditional layouts did not always meet the needs of certain situations. At such times, I began to design my own layouts, making, for example, cards 1, 2, 3, and 4 stand for a client's job prospects and cards 5, 6, 7, and 8 stand for that person's love life. These readings were as accurate and as satisfactory as the readings I did with more conventional layouts. What I was doing, before I began, was establishing a new meaning for my symbols, and so redefining the way I viewed reality.

There seems to be a natural law here that allows such changes to occur, but only if the new system is agreed upon before we begin to act upon the symbols. Thus, what did not work was to change the definitions of the card patterns halfway through the reading. If, after turning over cards 1 and 2, I decided that they should really represent someone's love life, the whole exercise would be meaningless, offering only garbled results. At that point, I would have to start all over again, reshuffling the cards and deciding what layout and meanings I wanted to use.

Any system of symbols works when everyone agrees on it ahead of time and then agrees to function within that system. This is especially true when designing ceremonies and rituals. With that knowledge, the next question to answer is what system to choose. A set of beliefs and symbols is an essential framework for any ritual practice, but how to make that decision?

There are three different methods that I use to design a symbol system for a ritual.

1) The personalized-symbol method
2) The culturally-rooted method
3) The mix-and-match method

THE PERSONALIZED-SYMBOL Method

What I mean by the personalized-symbol method is that the system a group or individual creates is based on their personal beliefs or experiences. A good example of this in an everyday context is the secret language that some twins develop among themselves. To an outsider the language may sound unintelligible or meaningless, but to the two that understand its code it can convey a complexity of shared meaning. Married couples or old friends often develop a vocabulary of private jokes, subtle gestures, and oblique references to shared experiences that they can use to communicate with each other without spectators understanding.

Even when using the same language as the people around us, various misunderstandings may arise because, for each of us, our life experiences have given us different personal associations for words that we share in common. To illustrate this point: I remember overhearing a conversation between a young white woman and an older Native man. They were talking about the ceremony of the vision-quest, in which the seeker fasts for a number of days while praying for guidance from the spirit realm.

After listening for a while, I could see that even though they were both speaking English, they were having trouble communicating because, without knowing it, they had different meanings for the verb "to fast." To the young woman, "to fast" meant to go without food only. This meant she could still consider herself to be fasting while she was living on water and juices, often for weeks at a time. To the Native man, "to fast" meant to go without food and water for a limited time for the purpose of prayer; naturally, it is not normally possible to fast, in this sense, for weeks at a time. When I explained to them how they perceived the same English word differently, they could come to an agreement in their discussion.

We unknowingly run across this type of communication problem all the time in our daily lives, but when we come together to perform ritual these communication difficulties take on an added significance because, in order to do effective group ritual, the members must share similar meanings for most of the concepts (including language symbols) that they use. Such commonality of meaning takes time and many shared experiences to develop, which can present problems for groups wishing to bond together quickly.

Many people have very deep feelings about their spirituality and their connection to the Earth. They don't know how to communicate their feelings to others in words, because the English language is very limited in its spiritual and emotional vocabulary. This is all right as long as they work solo, but if they want to work with a group they need a common set of symbols and a way to talk about their feelings.

With the personalized-symbol method, there is a lot of room for creativity and personal expression, but it also has certain limitations. A ritual practice based on a personal system relies so exclusively on the power of the individual or the group that it can have only as much power as the group or individual has to give at a particular time.

This can mean a lack of consistency. One ritual may be very powerful, while the next is only mediocre. Over time, it will be difficult to count on the effectiveness of your rites, and so you may become disillusioned and feel that the whole process is a meaningless exercise, and therefore give up entirely.

This is not to deny the power in personal symbols. Most of my personal ritual items are charged with my own power and intent, and so work well for me. They have deep significance to me, but they might not work for another person.

There is an exercise I do with my students in which I ask them to create for themselves a personal medicine wheel out of whatever materials they choose. This is a sacred circle, with four directional colors and other symbols associated with each of the four compass points. I am always amazed at how beautiful these creations can be, but sometimes I also mentally cringe at some of the colour and object combinations that my students design.

To me, these unfamiliar patterns seem wrong and out of alignment. When I question the students more closely about why they made what they did, I find they usually have a good reason that makes perfect sense when viewed from their perspectives. Even though those medicine wheels wouldn't work for me, they work perfectly well for the students who created them out of their own personal associations, so they are as valid for their creators' personal work as any wheel I could make would be for me.

THE CULTURALLY-ROOTED Method

The second method of choosing a ritual symbol system allows the student to pick a cultural system and then totally immerse oneself in that milieu. To use this method takes a lot of study and hard work, and those who seriously study a spiritual path for a number of years usually settle on one particular system for their work. Often practitioners who have used a personal symbol system for some time choose to deepen their practice by immersing themselves in the system of a particular culture that they are especially drawn to.

Most people of European origins, both in Europe and North America, are in ignorance of the Pagan past of their own ancestors, and have chosen to study with teachers of either Native American or Asian philosophies. This path has been a very satisfying one for many, but in my opinion, any person choosing a system in which he or she has no cultural or genetic roots is at a big disadvantage. Many would argue that this is not so, but I feel that there is a genetic link that taps us into racial memories that we can't find any other way.

In debating this issue with friends, I have found that there are several points that are usually brought up. One is, what if you are from a variety of genetic backgrounds? How do you choose which system to study? Not an easy question. I would answer, that by meditation over time, you will find the path that resonates right for you. Often students resist being totally open to the guidance of the inner self in this matter, because they have already decided that a certain path is the "right way" for them. A lot of white people resist studying their own roots, because they have romantic notions that other races are more spiritual or noble than they are. It's also harder to find out about the Pagan past of many European cultures, because it has been buried by the imperialistic Christian churches colonial practices for so many centuries.

I can sympathize with people who resist studying their European roots, because I did the same thing. When I was in my twenties and well into my Native studies, I had a dream in which I was told that I should speak for the Old Ones of my European heritage. At the time I knew nothing of Wicca. I totally rebelled, and resisted exploring my Celtic roots for many years after that, unwilling to let go of the Native way that was so clear to me, in order to search for another, less-trodden path.

I see people flocking to the Native way all the time. They know little of their own roots, yet seek fulfilment from a culture to which they have little connection. I have known people who over time, and I mean many years, have been able to establish a strong connection with a spiritual path that they are not racially or culturally connected to, and that's okay, but I believe that they will never feel entirely complete if they only know their adopted way and never experience their roots.

What if your genetic background truly doesn't resonate to you? I have a friend who is Jewish, and feels that she doesn't have any Pagan past, so what is she to do? I told her to be creative, and have suggested that she might study the past of the Middle East, and in particular Sumer, which was at one time conquered by Jews, with many Sumerian women taken as brides. Compromises of this sort are possible, but try to be creative and explore the past you know of from another perspective first.

She also knows that she had Jewish ancestors from Germany and Russia, and she feels drawn to the Norse tradition. Scandinavia is, of course, bracketed by Germany and Russia, and, considering the way Jews were often involuntarily moved from one part of Europe to another, she may indeed have ancestors who lived in Scandinavia at one time. And today there is always DNA testing to pin down your biological heritage if you need to personally clarify a connection. If we go back far enough, all of us have Pagan roots, although they may not be well documented.

The next thing that always comes up is the argument that you were a member of that group in another lifetime, and so have a strong need to re-establish that connection. I would not dream of putting myself in a position to say whether someone's past-life regressions are correct or not, but I would suggest that what happened in a past life is just that, a past life. You did that and it's over, and now it's time to deal with the challenges of this lifetime. So, for example, if in this life you were born European, then your challenge is to experience that life-essence fully, not try to return to another time when you were a part of another culture.

What I often find when talking to a person who claims to have been a Native medicine man or woman in another life is that the memories of that life are usually quite vague. What I think is actually happening is that such a person is very sensitive to the call of the land itself, and this desire to reconnect with the Earth is what is really beneath the desire to identify with a particular racial or cultural group to which one does not belong. If a person has such feelings but lacks a structure to express them, it is easy to gravitate to the Native way, but I argue that sometimes "easy" may be too easy.

If you are European, your challenge in this lifetime is to find a European way to serve the land. I honor those people for their sensitivity, but I suggest that they take the time to really pray about what is their true reason to be born at this time with those feelings. It is a difficult path, but European peoples around the world urgently need to re-establish their connections with the Earth, and teachers and leaders who are willing to make that commitment are desperately needed if we are to survive as a species.

In particular, I believe what is needed is a revival of the Goddess-centered, Earth-worshipping Pagan legacy, more than the cult of the warrior, which exists in, for instance, the Japanese, the Norse, the Hindu, and some Native cultures. So dig deeper, and find the female-centered as well as the male-centered traditions.

There is a valid need for immigrant peoples to this continent to create for themselves a spiritual link with this land on which they now live, but that must be done with a feeling of pride and self-worth, not guilt. No one can give another a feeling of self-worth and pride in one's heritage. No matter how much of an affinity you feel for the Native way, if you as a non-Native choose to walk the Native path, then come to your adopted people from a place of strength and self-respect. Take the time to learn about the Old Religions of your biological heritage—prior to Christian, Islamic or other colonialization; they are your cultural and racial birthright. Then seek out Native elders to teach you how to honor the Earth and the spirits of the land that is now your adopted home.

⚜

THE MIX-AND-MATCH METHOD

Using ritual and mythological materials from a number of different culture sources and time periods is the approach usually adopted by most ritual groups living in the U.S. and Canada today. Most modern Pagans living in these countries have only a superficial knowledge of their spiritual past. Those who use this system do so with the justification that everything is a part of the "one universal truth," so it is okay to blend the use of Gods and Goddesses and other symbols with little regard for their meaning within their original cultural context.

I personally find this type of system workable but a bit chaotic, and over a long period of time lacking in real depth for the serious student. The mix-and-match method works best for people who see their spirituality as a part of their life, rather than as a way of life. They have no time for the intense study necessary to follow a culturally-rooted method, and the deep commitment needed to be a Pagan priest or priestess is not what they want; they want something that will make them feel good and enhance their lives. Many people wish to follow a Pagan way as an alternative to their Judeo-Christian upbringing, and they want the Pagan rituals to occupy about the same proportion of their lives as the church or synagogue did in their childhoods. For them, the mix-and-match method works perfectly.

Do we need to break down "European" traditions into their component parts? I have spoken in this book of the Celtic tradition, for example, but it actually consists primarily of three different cultures—the Scots, the Irish, and the Welsh. Norse mythology is closely linked with that of other Germanic cultures. The Roman Gods and Goddesses are almost identical to the Greek ones, under different names. The Jewish culture is spread over all of Europe, and can be divided roughly into the Sephardic and the Ashkenazic strains. There have been so many invasions, and so many mixings, that you're not going to find a culturally-pure heritage. So there is a good argument that anyone of European background is entitled to use any European tradition they feel drawn to. Another argument is that the important thing now is not to bother about the past, but use whatever we wish to create the ceremonies we need for the future.

This mixing seems to be a condition of the North American experience which to some extent is unavoidable. There is little cultural material from the past for most of us to draw upon (even for many Native groups that have lost most of their cultural heritage), and as yet most immigrants to this land lack a deep connection with the land itself. So we do the best we can with what we have, and over time, both personally and as a group, ceremonies will evolve to deepen our spiritual practices.

⚬⚬

SUMMARY:

I tend to see these three systems as interchangeable. All are applicable at different occasions or stages of personal or group development. For example, a group or individual may begin by working with a ritual symbol system that they have derived from a variety of sources. They may have read a few books or attended a number of workshops. From this material, they will put together a system that will get them started on their spiritual paths. As time goes on, the person or group may wish to concentrate their work in a particular cultural area, or they may wish to work with their own personalized system that has developed over time.

Even if they concentrate on one particular system, they may also use a different system when that seems most appropriate for a certain purpose. A friend says she can't imagine doing a ritual dealing with cats that doesn't invoke Bastet (or Sekhmet, the lion-goddess, for big cats), although she is not greatly drawn to Egyptian mythology in other ways.

Keep in mind that there is no right and wrong way here. It is only necessary to know that you do have choices as to what works best in a particular situation.

Understanding what you are doing and what your choices are makes it easier to create the system that works best for your group, and if circumstances change then you have the tools with which to adapt to meet the new challenge.

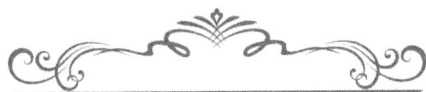

Chapter 7

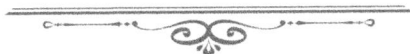

Some Thoughts about
Cultural Ownership and Honoring the Land

I was once invited to a talking-stick circle in a nearby city. The circle was made up of both Native and non-Native people who came together regularly to support each other and pray. The philosophical outlook of this group was basically Native with some European Pagan elements added on. During the evening I attended, the circle was interrupted by some Native people from one of the local bands. They were very unhappy about this circle's existence, and wanted to make their opinions known. The whole confrontation was very upsetting for everyone present, and at one point things got rather out of hand when shouts and accusations were exchanged.

As more and more urban people become aware of a need to rediscover a way of life that is in harmony with the Earth, they often look to Native people for that guidance, hoping the Natives will show them how to reclaim what they feel they have lost.

In their way, most of these people are very sincere in their desire to honor the Earth and the ancient Native traditions. However, many Natives find this interest very invasive or threatening, often with good reason from their perspective. These Natives see their spirituality as the last thing that the white man hasn't taken from them, and they are afraid that if they give it away now they will have nothing left.

Their views are strengthened when they see non-Natives who have studied for a short time with Native elders then go on to teach or write books about what they have learned, often collecting large profits for themselves while doing little to help out or acknowledge the people who taught them. I have heard this type of practice referred to as New Age imperialism.

I don't think the issue is quite as black-and-white as Native fundamentalists would like us to believe, but there are certainly good arguments to be considered on both sides. Somewhat simplified, it seems to me to be an issue of what does a particular people or culture own, and what belongs to the land itself and so can rightfully be used by anyone living upon that ground?

Similar types of ceremonies have sprung up in many parts of the world. These places are often far apart, so explaining the similarities as the exchange of ideas is hardly possible. The example that comes to mind as I write this is the sweat-lodge ceremony. For those not familiar with it, this is a Native North American ceremony where a small hut is built with a pit in the centre into which heated rocks are put. Participants go inside, the door is shut, and water is poured over the rocks, creating steam. The purpose of this rite is to cleanse oneself and to pray. As the sauna, the same rite is found in Northern Europe. The sauna is now usually a purely physical act, but it used to have a ritual meaning similar to that still existing among North American Natives. Something similar used to be done in Siberia also.

A sweat-lodge is usually performed with special songs and prayers that belong only to this type of ceremony. The songs and prayers will vary depending on what Native band performs the sweat, but I would argue that the idea of the sweat-lodge itself belongs to the land. So, what that means to me in practical terms is that, if I perform a sweat-lodge using songs and other cultural materials that belong to another racial or ethnic group, maybe they might have a right to be upset with me if they feel that they have not given me permission to use their materials. Think of it sort of like a violation of a cultural copyright.

It's a little like wearing a kilt if you're not Scottish, or wearing a dashiki if you're not African. These things must look, at best, pointless and, at worst, pretentious and boastful, to people who are ethnically entitled to do them.

On the other hand, if I feel directed to do a sweat and use materials that I develop myself, or that come from my racial and cultural background, then I have the right to get a little snarky if someone comes along and tells me to stop. In this case, the directive to do the ceremony is coming from the Earth Mother herself, and is available to all her children who live on the type of land where variants of this ceremony are appropriate. I know there are many who would disagree with my conclusions, but I believe they help to explain why, for the first time in many centuries, so many people are being drawn to create and perform ceremonies that are not a part of the cultural tradition in which they were raised. I believe, that as threats of global destruction increase, the Earth is calling to her more sensitive children to recreate for themselves the Earth-related ancient rites.

The issue can be more complicated than this. For example, many Natives have a deep reverence for the sacred pipe or for smudges like sage or sweet-grass. They feel that these things need to be treated with the deepest respect, and they feel they have been "given" certain rules on how to behave when using these sacred objects. Modern non-Natives who have grown up in homes where only a superficial respect was paid to the Sacred often do things with these sacred objects out of ignorance (like buying or selling them in stores) that make more knowledgeable people very angry. After all, how do patriotic Americans feel when they see Natives wearing an upside-down U.S. flag on their ceremonial regalia? This is a violation of American law, just as buying or selling sweet-grass is a violation of Native spiritual codes.

As a further illustration, I recall seeing a young Australian (white) man playing a didgeridoo at a gathering. The sound sent shivers down my back. I could feel the power in that ancient music from down under. The sound was a very potent male essence that added a lot to the ritual that was performed that night, but later, sitting around the fire, this man let a lot of people play with the instrument in very irreverent ways and for very unspiritual motives.

After talking to this young man, I found him to be a very sincere man searching for a path and trying, most of the time, to do the right thing. The problem, as I saw it, was that he had bought the didgeridoo at a store and hadn't taken the time to really understand and get to know, in a sacred way, the instrument he now owned, before he started taking it to rituals.

I have met so many people in my travels like this young man. They feel the call of the Earth but lack the skills, and are not always willing to take the time to learn properly, how to honor the visions that they have been shown.

So after saying all that one might ask, "Okay, how do I learn about the Earth and care for the Sacred?" I'm not sure I can offer you an easy formula, but I can offer some suggestions as to where to look for your own answers.

For those of you growing up with few cultural roots and little or no attachment to the land on which you live, I would suggest that your task is two-fold. The first is to come to some sort of understanding of your cultural heritage, in the sense of finding out how your ancestors paid honor to the Earth and lived in harmony with the life around them. The second is to personally "get to know" the Earth in the area where you live. By combining your own culture with a sense of the land, you can create a personal or group ceremonial practice that will be creative and satisfying, and will aid in returning a sense of harmony and balance to the Earth.

You can begin to understand your cultural roots by studying books on the topic (though have a care for the accuracy of your sources), or you may be lucky enough to find a teacher wise in the ancient ways of your people from whom to learn. You can also tap into racial and cultural knowledge through dreams and consistent meditations on these topics. Satisfying results will not be gained overnight. They will take time and commitment over a long period, so be prepared for that and don't give up easily. Think of yourself as a hero on a quest – give in to the magic and mystery of it all.

The next step is to come to an understanding of the Earth and the guardian spirits of the land on which you live. If you are an urban dweller with little experience of the "bush," you probably harbor a fear of the wild untamed places, so it may be hard for you to take off to the wilds of the Rockies and feel comfortable there. Your fear may (unconsciously or consciously) get in the way of any true communication between you and the spirits of the Earth in that place.

For such a person, I would suggest that you take it slow. Begin at home with a garden in your backyard or with walks by the seashore or in a big city park. Never forget that, even under all the concrete and steel, the Earth still remains. It is not so glamourous and may take more time and effort, but there are still things of value to be found wherever you live. I have friends who dedicate a portion of their gardens to the Nature spirits and feel a lot of power emanating from that bit of Earth even though it is in the heart of a big city. Much of the literature written about Findhorn will give you valuable information on how to be in touch with the Nature spirits from a European perspective. This suggestion is not an endorsement of Findhorn, but there are ideas of value to be gained from their teachings.

For those who live in, or feel more comfortable with, the wilder places of this planet, I would recommend exploring the feel of the land in more natural settings. When you are travelling in the wild places, the idea is to listen to what the land has to tell you. This means you don't use the quiet of the woods to replay old tapes in your head of all your worldly problems. The aim is to try to turn off that internal dialogue so that you can learn to sense what is around you.

The purpose of your explorations is to find a suitable site for doing personal or group ceremonies. To discover one, you must find a place you can visit frequently, so that you can get to know it intimately in all its seasons. Such a ceremonial site can offer great wisdom and power, but to find that place you must know how to feel what is right for you.

The Earth is not all sweetness and light; there are places where people are most unwelcome at this time in our planet's herstory. Let me give a personal example. Some time ago, I had a relative set up a bush camp for me in a wilderness area not too far from the city in which I was then living. Logically speaking, to a man who was not too sensitive to the deeper spiritual aspects of the land, the site he chose was a good one. It was in a little clearing off the beaten path, near fresh water and among tall trees that broke the wind and rain coming off the ocean.

Physically, it was a beautiful spot to look at, but it was also a very disturbed place. Nearby there was a raw clear-cut, and between my camp and the cut lived something that was not sure it wanted any humans around for any reason. When I first tried to stay there, I took note of the occasional unreasonable feeling of fear that I had, especially near nightfall and coming from one particular place on the hillside above the camp. I didn't panic, nor did I ignore these feelings. I chose at first merely to take note of what was being sent to me, and see what needed to be done about it.

In time I gained an uneasy truce with the being at the top of the hill. I recognized that it had been sent to protect what was left of the old-growth forest there from anyone wishing to destroy more of the trees. I gained the truce by going there many times and staying for short visits. I set up an altar to the spirits of the place, and left offerings for the small woods creatures upon it.

As I write this, the best way I can think of to describe how I went about this work would be to liken the experience to how I would get to know and tame a wild animal. I took it slow. I didn't rush in to do a big ritual. I gave the Land time to taste and absorb my bodily essence, my blood, my piss, my shit. I gave the Land time to get to know and feel my energy in a quiet non-threatening way. Making no demands, I simply went there and allowed things to progress as they would.

When I felt the fear, I first had to decide that there was no actual physical danger present, like a cougar nearby. When I felt that my physical safety was assured, I acknowledged the sending that was being given, but I didn't act upon it. I went on with my camp chores or went for a walk till things cooled down.

I passed several seasons in this manner, but though I was tolerated there I never felt it was a place of sanctuary and power for me. This land had been too deeply wounded to have any energy left over to help humankind. There are many places on our planet that are now like this, so you may need time to search to find an ideal spot that will be open to you establishing a psychic/spiritual link with it.

To cite a more positive example, I recall a year spent living in a small cabin by a woodland lake. During my stay there, I feel I developed a deep connection with the spirit that lived in that lake. I began getting to know the lake by trying to spend some time each day alone, swimming or kayaking on the lake. I swam each day until late fall, even though there was snow on the ground some days and the water was very cold. I felt very loved and protected by that lake. I would describe the water as sensuously cool rather than cold.

In the cooler months I didn't stay in as long as in the summer when I swam across the lake, but I did go in and swim out into deep water for more than just a dip and out again—like the New Year's Polar Bear Swim. These swims were usually at about the same time each day. It got to the point that I could hear the lake calling to me even while I was busy elsewhere or visiting with friends. When I felt this call, I would look at a clock and know it was about the time I usually went in. I was given a lot of gifts that year from the lake – things that are too personal to talk about here, but they did change me, and from that came a deeper understanding and power for which I am very grateful.

Before leaving this topic, I would like to suggest that, for many of us, not only bush skills and time, but a change in how we view the land is important. Unconsciously, often, many people (especially men) view their spiritual training as a test. They need to be strong and overcome pain or discomfort to be worthy. That type of thinking has a place, but it is not the only way.

To go back to the lake example, at the same time I was swimming the lake, a man down the road was doing the same thing. He would swim the lake every day just as I did, but he saw his experience in a totally different light. For him, the lake was very cold. He saw his swim as an ordeal. He saw the lake as something he needed to conquer to make himself worthy and strong, so he could be blessed by spiritual insights. I was surprised when he told me how cold he found the lake, because I had hardly noticed it at all. I don't feel that I am tougher than this fellow, but my attitude was very different, so my experience was as well. To me, the lake was a mother welcoming a lost child home, not a being to be conquered. I suggest that sometimes to "make love" to the land is a wiser approach than it is to try to change or conquer it. This is where woman's wisdom will often gain you more understanding than some of the old male beliefs, from any tradition you choose.

The connection that a group or individual establishes with the land may be a cultural one or it may be a deeply personal one. There are places on this continent where non-Native peoples have connected very deeply with Earth spirits in an area. Their Native neighbors may call the spirits by different names (according to what was given to their cultures), but the energy behind the name is the same. The name used by each people is equally valid; it's the spiritual connection that is what will bring about the healing of our planet, not the parroting of old cultural patterns from whatever background.

One last point to note when trying to re-create a connection with the land to establish ceremony. It is possible to invite Gods or Goddesses or spirits from another part of the world, but to whom you feel connected, to come be a part of your practice in a new area where they may not have been known before. There are parts of the Eastern coast where, after almost five hundred years, the integration between the Native and the old European deities can be felt. This is a goal toward which I hope we all can work, so that in the future an integrated ceremonial system will be there to meet the needs of all of us living on this continent.

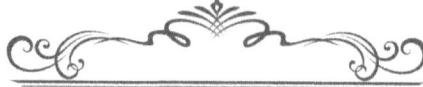

Chapter 8

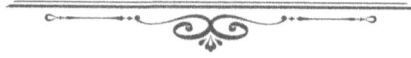

The Backbone of Ritual

During the 1970's, when I was in graduate school, I became quite involved in local Native politics. Along with all the sit-ins and other protests, I can remember long hours spent with friends discussing the pros and cons of Native versus modern white society. As I recall, the merits of our Native culture far surpassed anything coming out of Europe. We behaved quite cruelly towards our non-Native friends and justified our behavior, at least to ourselves, by the feeling that "they" deserved it because of how "we" had been treated by whites for over four hundred years. White people were always asking stupid questions and their scientists were destroying the Earth—so we said then.

Looking back now, I have to sigh with regret at my ignorance, because behind this mask of haughty superiority was the face of self-hatred and pain. I am Metis, a mixed blood. I look more white than Native. To act the way I did was to deny the reality of myself. I lived in such a black-and-white reality back then. Native culture was so good (at least the old medicine ways), and white culture was so bad. If I identified with my white self, the bad culture, then I would be bad myself, so in desperation I clung to my illusions to keep from killing myself.

Years later, when I discovered Wicca, I found that positive image of white society that I had been looking for. I now strongly believe that no one people have a monopoly on "the way." Prejudice and romantic idealization of a people are two sides of the same coin. (The Drunken Indian and the Noble Savage are equally harmful to the people thus stigmatized.) Each people and culture on this planet were given part of the ancient Wisdom, and all must be brought together to create a balanced, healthy world.

Through meditation, I was guided to see that, like the eagle they honor, Native traditions take a large over-view of life. The Native way, like all indigenous cultural traditions, is intuitive and experiential. These old Earth-rooted cultures see things in whole units and broad perspectives, but that is only one point on the wheel of life.

The scientific-technological attitude is a polar opposite to the indigenous world-view. Scientists are always analyzing and dissecting the world around them. In its earliest stages, this method produces ignorance and destruction of the worst kind. But taken to its logical conclusions, as is now happening in the field of quantum physics, the beliefs of theoretical physicists and cosmologists have begun to converge with the long-held faith of the medicine man.

One of the things that modern techno-society has to offer the "spiritual wheel" of ancient tradition is its ability to ask questions. Many Natives believe that if they ask questions and analyze their religion, it will lose its power. This, I believe, is not true. To be able to understand why some things work and to be able to take them apart and put them back together is a valuable skill, both in the physical and the spiritual world. It is not a curse. In the Native tradition, there are some very powerful and beautiful rites, but sometimes these rituals can be uncompromisingly static and unable to adapt to new situations. Time and time again, the young are told, "We do it this way because that is how we do it and don't ask questions."

The problem with this kind of reasoning is that rituals must change with the times or they will no longer meet the needs of their people. To some extent, that is what is happening in many indigenous communities today. Young people growing up in a modern world with school and TV and alcoholism see little connection between their lives and these rites that cling to a vanished past.

I am not advising throwing out the old ways; far from it. I am merely saying that at this time in our history, more, perhaps, than at any other, we need to ask "why?" This is where the teachings of the scientist can help. If we can ask of a ceremony "What in your performance brings in the power, what are the pieces of the pattern, why does it work this way and not when we do this instead?" – if we can find out this type of information, then we can break down a ritual to the essence of its parts and re-create it again in the same or in a new form to meet different circumstances, yet still contain all the power of the original rite. Then we truly have a rite of power that will meet our needs today and those of our children in generations to come.

From these musings began my search to find the magic building blocks, the parts that would be common to most ceremonies. I reasoned that, with such building blocks, we could re-create the ceremonies to meet our changing needs. From my studies, I came up with an idea I call my "cakeness" theory of ritual structure. A very "feminine" musing, but let me explain.

Suppose I have a recipe that has been handed down through my family for generations telling how to make a cake. My recipe is for chocolate cake, good chocolate cake. One problem, however, is that my recipe tells me how to make only one kind of cake – chocolate. With this recipe I am limited, but it works, so I am happy and I pass this wonderful recipe on to my children. This is how most people experience life. They follow in the footsteps of their ancestors, and as long as they follow the pattern they feel secure, and everything is right with their world. This works only as long as the conditions in the outside world do not change.

Getting back to "cakeness": if my grandchildren, for example, cannot obtain chocolate for their cakes because some outside circumstance causes chocolate to be unavailable, then they have a real problem. In this case, to cling to a chocolate cake recipe when there is no chocolate will probably create a lot of stress. But cakes are wonderful treats, and my grandchildren cannot bear to give them up entirely. The solution? If my honorable descendants can discover the principle of "cakeness," they will know what to do. If they discover that flour, sugar, eggs, and fat of some kind are common to all cake recipes, they can change with the times. With these ingredients and a few added ones now available instead of chocolate, they can make spice, pineapple, or banana cake, and all these varieties will be just as delicious as the old chocolate cake, because they all have the same basic ingredients in common.

These principles are true for ritual as well. If you can find the pieces of the pattern that all, or at least most, successful rituals have in common, then, even though you may not possess a handed-down formula, you can still have a workable, powerful ceremonial system.

There is a hidden danger in this method, however. Analysis of ritual must be balanced with experience or the whole process becomes a meaningless intellectual exercise. Balancing the teachings of the scientist and the shaman is perhaps the challenge of our time.

Part of my university training included a BA in cultural anthropology. As I studied my course material, I gained insights into religious practices around the world. Later when I began to study the spiritual process in our modern Pagan communities, my nearly-forgotten study techniques came in handy. Combining my training with the knowledge I had as a practicing Pagan ceremonialist, I began to look at what steps in the ceremonial process are common to most cultures around the world.

The Seven Steps discussed in the second half of this book are what I have found to be common to successful rituals in most cultures. These building blocks of ceremony are listed here and discussed in more detail in Part Two of this book. The Steps are guidelines only. Each group of people is expected to choose the activities within the Steps that best meet the needs of their community practice.

The activities and the time and care put into preparing them will determine the success and flavor of the work. But the Seven Steps, in some form, should always make up the backbone of the ritual work. There are endless possibilities. Through study, the teachings of your elders, and your own group's creativity it is possible to create a dynamic ceremonial system that will be powerful and fulfilling.

❧

THE SEVEN BASIC STEPS of Ritual

Step 1: The Planning of a Ceremony

Deciding what will be done and who will do it, where and when and who will be there, and any other practical details.

❧

STEP 2: THE PREPARATION of a Ceremony

A. Doing the inner work and psychological preparation.

B. Gathering costumes, masks and other personal adornments.

C. Gathering tools, props and sacred items for the altar.

D. Practicing sacred theatre.

❧

STEP 3: CREATING SACRED Space

    A. Cleaning the location.

    B. Arranging the altars and other gear.

STEP 4: THE CLEANSING and Blessing

    A. Purifying the site.

    B. Purifying the people.

STEP 5: THE OPENING of the Ritual

    A. Creating sacred space – the circle.

    B. Invoking the deities – prayer.

    C. Stating the intention of the ritual.

    Step 6: The Body of the Ritual

    A. Creating the sound field – music and song.

    B. Dancing.

    C. Performing sacred theatre.

    D. Other – guided visualization, talking-stick circles, the give-away ceremony, cone of power.

STEP 7: THE CONCLUSION of the Ritual

    A. Saying farewell to the deities and thanking them.

    B. Grounding the participants.

    C. Enjoying the feast.

    D. Cleaning the site.

    E. Storing the ritual items.

    F. Processing the effects of the ritual on the participants.

THE SUBTOPICS ARE ONLY suggestions; few rituals will include everything listed above. However, any successful ritual needs to include something from each of the Seven Steps.

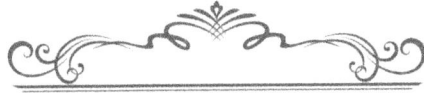

PART TWO

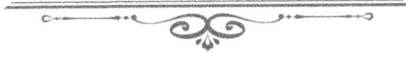

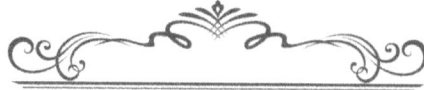

Chapter 1

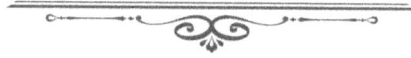

Step 1:
Ceremony Planning

Somewhere in the far beyond, the essence of a ritual is conceived. It drifts there, in the void, timeless, formless, waiting for the mind of humankind to touch its being and bring it forth into the reality of the physical plane. And so it begins. Someone feels inspired to do a ceremony. At first it may not be clear what type of ceremony, but over time the ideas and images will become clearer and clearer until they emerge fully formed into our physical reality.

I'd like to begin with a few comments, then end this section with some basic outlines for seasonal rites lasting for more than two days' duration.

Let me state once again that the focus of this section is on the seasonal community rite lasting for two or more days. There are other good books on the market that can help you plan an evening's event for those who wish to honor the seasonal energies, yet are too busy with other projects to spend a lot of time in preparing for, or participating in, a long ceremonial event. For those with the inclination, I hope this section will give you some suggestions to use in creating your own ceremonial system.

Though it has often been frustrating for me to acknowledge it, I have come to accept that not everyone has the same need for long rituals in their lives. The question, as I see it, is to decide for yourself if ceremony is to be a part of your life, or a way of life. In the former case, ritual will be something done occasionally to honor the Sacred and to (hopefully) come away from the rite with pleasant feelings of contentment and renewal. This is a perfectly valid way to approach the Sacred, and it requires only a minimum of planning and preparation.

For others, however, this may not be enough, either because they have grown up in a tradition that demands more of them, or because by doing simpler rituals they have acquired a desire to go deeper into the ceremonial experience.

When working in groups to do ritual, it is important to clarify where members stand on this issue. Often group members have different expectations of the ritual process and do not understand each other's needs. This can lead to countless misunderstandings and hurt feelings when these differences surface later during group rites. If all members can agree that they wish to participate in the longer ceremonial process and are willing to put in the necessary time (often months) needed to achieve the best results, then the event will most likely be successful and satisfying for all. The ritual process, as I practice it, begins with a core group of six or more people who gather regularly to plan a community ritual event. Four of these people become what I call the "clan leaders;" this is a term that is appropriate in the particular ceremonial system I use. I will explain it in detail in Chapter Two. What is important here is that there be a core group willing to dedicate time to preparing the ceremony; the process used to allocate tasks is up to you.

Ideally, members should begin their meetings two or three months ahead of time to plan and prepare for the ceremony. This may seem like a long time, but it is necessary if the event is to be a ceremony that will include many segments and last longer than a few hours of an evening. The power of the rite needs time to grow and mature. As the participants focus their energies more and more upon the ritual to come, the power of that rite will build into a strong transforming force that can make real changes in the lives of the people who are attending the event.

My main focus is on the seasonal event, but before giving some examples of that, let me discuss briefly other reasons for performing sacred rites.

⚜

RITES OF PASSAGE

Life experiences that crave the celebration of ritual include births, deaths, marriages and puberty rites. These are often incorporated into seasonal ceremonies, and that may be appropriate, but I tend to treat these events as separate from seasonal rites. I was taught to view them this way by my elders because usually, in my tradition, these events are sponsored by a particular person or family within a community and so are planned and directed by that sponsor rather than by the community itself. As with any event, the more time and energy put into the planning and preparation, the more powerful the rite is likely to be.

The time spent helps prepare the psyche for changes in one's life after a major passage. There is not always an opportunity to prepare for a death, and we are not used to celebrating coming-of-age, but even in our modern culture, we spend a great deal of time and effort in preparing for births and marriages. I refer to such things as baby showers, choosing names, planning elaborate weddings, countless fittings of bridal dresses, planning honeymoons, etc. All of this is the modern way of focusing our mental and physical energies on an important event to come. When we as Pagans spend a long time planning a seasonal ritual, we focus our energies on an event in a similar way.

HEALING RITUALS

The other type of ritual that is often performed during a seasonal ceremony is a healing ritual. If the work is for the group as a whole, then appropriate healing exercises can be planned. I'm thinking here of guided visualizations and other process work that can be done by the entire group in an evening. They can be done during full or new Moon rituals as well as during seasonal rites. Over time, these process-oriented exercises can achieve very powerful results. I use and recommend them when group members cannot allot a single large block of time to do the necessary healing.

For someone who is emotionally or physically ill, the traditional method in many cultures was to have an entire healing ceremony focusing on that person and his or her problem. In such a case, the healing of the person becomes the sole focus for the ceremony. Such rituals usually last for several days—24 hours of those several days. During the event one or more healers will concentrate their energies and that of the group itself towards the healing of the individual for whom the ceremony has been called.

I prefer not to explain this type of ceremony in much detail, because I feel quite strongly that these rituals should not be attempted by unskilled people and so are beyond the scope of this present writing, but I do feel they have a place in our future ceremonial systems. Briefly, what happens is this. The ceremony begins by opening the patient's awareness to previously unthought-of aspects and dimensions of the illness. Several healers work together with supportive friends and family members to raise and maintain an energy field that will aid in the patient's healing.

They work on the issue at hand for many days. When the process is complete, they close and ground the work and bring about a feeling of unity and solidarity among all present that will help support the patient in an ongoing way after the ceremony has been completed. If you are not familiar with the type of rite I am referring to, there are countless descriptions of it in anthropological accounts.

To offer a more modern example from the New Age, I remember a friend telling me about a one-day ceremony held for him a few years back. The doctor had diagnosed a tumor and had scheduled him for an operation one week later. During that time, his wife, who was a Reiki practitioner, gathered together a number of friends and Reiki healers. The ritual was relatively unstructured, with a lot of fun being had by all, but for 24 hours straight one or more people were doing hands-on healing focused on my friend's body. The result of this ritual was that when he went in to have the surgery the doctors could find no trace of the tumor. I am not advocating ritual as the sole alternative to modern medicine, but I do feel that there is room to explore how long ceremonies can enhance other forms of treatment.

I see advantages to the ritual method, especially in the area of psychology. For example, if a person has an old childhood trauma (like incest) to deal with, the usual method is to see a therapist of some type, often for years at a time. If something that is very upsetting comes up during a weekly session, when the allotted time is over the client is supposed to leave, often with his emotional guts hanging out, because there is another patient waiting to be seen.

In a ceremony this would not happen. The work would continue until it had come to some type of natural conclusion. The patient would then be given a chance to ground himself, so that when he returned to the everyday world there would be some sort of conclusion to the process that would allow him or her to function normally. This is not to say that the same issue cannot be treated at another time, but after the rituals, if done properly, the individual should be able to live life normally and with a sense of well-being. I hope that, in future,

New Age practitioners will explore this method of treatment further, because I feel it has a lot to offer our modern world.

SEASONAL RITES

Returning once more to our original topic of seasonal rituals, I want to start with a few comments. First of all, I stress taking lots of time in planning and preparing for ceremonial events, but realistically no one person or group can prepare for every seasonal rite in detail. Most spiritual systems around the world have from five to nine seasonal events within a year's cycle. That is just too many for anyone to give full attention to. Even among societies where ritual is a way of life, different families or parts of the community take responsibility for different events. They divide up the year so that the burden falls equally on everyone.

No matter what your belief system is, whether Native, Christian, Hindu, or Pagan, all religions have seasonal celebrations. Traditionally, the reason for doing seasonal rituals was to preserve and heal the Earth and "keep it going"—some traditions actually believe the Spring will not come if they don't do their Spring rituals, for instance. Other traditions, and most modern groups, don't take seasonal rituals quite so literally, but they still do retain aspects of these ancient beliefs.

I am working in an adapted Celtic system of ceremony, with eight seasonal holidays, but the principles I describe here can be applied to other religious systems. My seasonal rituals incorporate inner work by the participants, along with celebrating agricultural festivals. I do this in order to integrate human beings (especially urban dwellers) back into the natural cycle of the Earth.

If your group is new at this type of experience, I would recommend that you begin with one seasonal event, then work up to no more than four major events in a yearly cycle. I don't mean to imply that you do not honor the other seasons simply that you celebrate them less elaborately for the year or attend someone else's planned event. As a personal preference, I tend to like to plan longer ceremonies to celebrate the Pagan cross-quarter days of Samhain (October 31 - November 1), Imbolg (February 1 - 2), Beltane (April 30 - May

1), and Lughnasadh (July 31 - August 1), while honoring the solstices and equinoxes in a quieter fashion.

My reasoning for this relates to the fact that I feel the cross-quarter days are more Earth-centered, female-centered holidays, rather than the solar, male-centered rituals of the Sun cycle. At the cross-quarter days in the climate of the northern hemisphere in which I live, I sense a shift in the universal energy flow that I don't feel at the solstices and equinoxes.

Perhaps this is because in the old days the dates of the cross-quarter ceremonies were reckoned by the phases and cycles of the Moon, and thus were celebrated more by the peasants and common folk than by the nobility. To determine the dates of the solstices and equinoxes needs a high degree of mathematical skill that could only have been achieved in earlier times by an educated elite, and so I believe the solstice and equinox rites were not connected as closely to the land itself.

As I said before, this is my own preference. For a long time, I only focused on the Samhain event because I felt the strongest connection with it. From that beginning I have tried to create a working system for each of the other three cross-quarter days that connects them together and enhances the power of each one. With the purpose of a yearly balance in mind, I use the following as my focus for the four events.

Samhain (October 31 - November 1) – The old Celtic New Year:

This is a time in our Northern climates when the harvest is over and all life is settling down to endure the long months of Winter's cold. It is a time for sitting by the fire with a good book or catching up on old projects that we had no time to finish in the warmer, more active months. This is also a time when the veil between the Worlds of the Living and the Dead is thinnest. The Underworld calls to us to look within ourselves for the answers to life's problems. It is wise at this season to honor our ancestors and seek counsel from our beloved dead. It is a time of pale, ghostly Moons and bonfires burning bright in the frosty night air. Modern society celebrates this occasion with costume parties and trick-or-treat, a sad echo of more ancient rites.

In the ceremonial system that I use, this is the time to present sacred theatre centered around a descent into the Underworld. During these rites, participants ask themselves, "What part of my life do I need to let go of? What is not functioning well for me? What do I need to change in the New Year to become a more healthy, balanced person?" The same questions can also apply to communities and to the land itself. Samhain is a time to look without fear at death and dying, and, during the winter, work on what will be born anew with the spring.

Imbolg (February 1 - 2) the word means in the belly:

This rite focuses on conception and creativity. The sacred theatre at this time would ask, "What gifts of understanding have I been given over the Winter, and, from this understanding, what is growing inside me?" This is a time of story-telling, poetry, and song. It is a time of new beginnings, seed plantings, and the idea stage of projects that will come to completion later in the year. This festival draws upon the energies of the Maiden Goddesses. If the group is an all-women's group, it is a good time to work with Blood mysteries. Men's groups may choose to explore the feminine side of their natures through their rituals at this time. For the land, this is the time when the light grows stronger and the plants and animals feel the first stirrings of Spring.

Beltane (April 30 - May 1) Fertility and Flowering:

Of all the seasonal ceremonies, I feel this is the time for joyous celebration. In most parts of the Northern hemisphere the weather is beautiful by this time, and many plants are beginning to flower and sprout edible stems. Sacred theatre now asks us to look at the question of "How am I putting into action in my life the plans and changes that were conceived over the Winter?"

To our European ancestors in the past, Beltane was a festival of fertility and sexual license. It definitely is a time when sexual energies run high, but I would offer a word of caution against allowing those energies to become too dominant at a group ritual. It would be more productive to the community to sublimate the sexuality into group projects and activities – something that the group can get excited about and passionately care about doing.

When possible, I use a Maypole with long ribbons that we tie to the top of the pole. Dancers each hold a ribbon. They divide into two circles moving in opposite directions about the Maypole. They weave the ribbons down the pole, alternately lifting their ribbons over the head of a dancer going the other way and ducking under the ribbon of the next dancer. The ribbons symbolize our pledges of action in the coming season. The weaving dance gives energy to our commitment.

Beltane, in some traditions, marks the change from the dark to the light half of the year. Because of its place across the wheel of the year from Samhain, it is also a time when the veil between the Worlds of the Living and the Dead is thin. For this reason, in ancient times, fires were lit on the hilltops to protect animals and people from ghosts. In my rituals, I don't stress the aspects of the Underworld, but I do acknowledge their presence as we move on to the fertile season of the year.

Lughnasadh (July 31 - August 1) The First Harvest:

For some reason that I can't quite explain, Lughnasadh is the ceremony that I have participated in the least. August in our modern culture seems to be a time when many people take vacations or are busy in other ways that make it difficult to get a long, intensive ritual happening. I think it has to do with our experiences in school. As children, when August comes around, we suddenly realize that the Summer vacation is almost over, and we frantically try to spend as much time as possible playing. We are unwilling to commit to anything that feels at all like work. I've always regretted that, because August has the potential to be one of the richest seasonal times.

The land is beginning to retire from the vigorous growing cycle of Spring and early Summer. Lughnasadh is the first of the Harvest feasts. It is a time when what was conceived at Imbolg and put into action at Beltane should be ready for harvesting, now or soon. But this is also a time to be wary, because the harvest may not be totally in the barn; there is still the danger of drought or hailstorms or other disasters that may destroy all that has been achieved during the growing cycle so far.

Just as Imbolg is a strong female time, I see Lughnasadh as a strong time of the male energies. It is the time when the man who chooses to be the guardian and warrior and protector of women, children, and the Earth herself needs to be honored and encouraged. In women's groups, the protective Mama Bear energy (or the Amazon warrior) is what should be aroused and channeled at this time.

In the sacred theatre of Lughnasadh, the questions are, "What have you harvested, and what from this experience needs to be kept safe and cherished?" This is a great time to do work around environmental issues, in keeping with the theme of protecting and restoring the Earth.

WHAT I HAVE JUST DISCUSSED are a few suggestions about how to create a workable interconnected system that will balance out the seasonal rites of the year, but bear in mind that this is but one system and it may or may not be appropriate for what you and your group choose to do. Other systems and traditions are equally valid as well.

The cross-quarter system described above was developed in the Northern hemisphere. I have never lived in the Southern hemisphere, but the few people I know who come from there tell me that Pagans in the South have two basic options. First, they can choose to follow their genetic heritage and celebrate the seasonal festivals as their ancestors did in Europe. Alternatively, they can develop a new system that is adapted to the seasons of the land where they live. This is for the Southern communities to decide.

The logical question that many people ask at this point is, "What do you do at a ceremony lasting days at a time?" For many who have not experienced it, the concept is more than a bit overwhelming. A long ceremonial is actually a series of smaller rituals and activities that are linked together by a particular theme and intent. At such an event, the energy tends to flow in waves, sometimes very exciting and active, at other times slow, dreamy, and meditative.

This is a natural progression that should be encouraged and worked with rather than ignored. Bear in mind, however, that you may lose the ritual's power and focus as the energies shift. Participants at first will need to be reminded to stay focused, even during breaks. Giving way to a lot of idle chatter may mean that it will be hard to get going again when breaks are over.

A word of warning: There is a tendency, when new at this work, to create a long ceremony by stringing together a series of unrelated events without a true sense of how they mesh together on deeper levels. This happens because most of us are trying to re-create what has been lost by drawing together bits and pieces from a variety of sources and traditions. These fragments are often not well understood, but what I feel is more important than collecting fragments of old rites is learning how to create new rites that preserve the essence of the old.

Let me cite a brief example. I was working once with a group that planned to hold a Beltane celebration. They had done some research and had a few ideas, two of which were jumping the Beltane fire and dancing around a May pole.

These two activities are very traditional in European Pagan practices, so would appear logical choices. The theme for this event was about how to channel sexuality into acts of creation rather than destruction in our lives.

When I questioned the group on how they planned to, logistically, use the May pole with forty or fifty untrained people, their answer was to have half the group weave the ribbons and the other half unweave them. This was what a local school did, and it shows how little deep understanding of the old ways often survives. This way of dancing a May pole would be fine for a children's game, but is not right for a serious magical ritual with intent. I was taught by my elders that the May pole symbolizes the binding of the wild energy of the male (which is loosed in the winter, with the Wild Hunt) so that this energy can be used in the spring to fertilize the Earth and all female-kind. In the fall, the same energy would be once more released by burning the May pole or unweaving the ribbons. So, to weave the pole and then unweave it during the same ritual would mean unweaving the magic just done.

This type of spell-casting also needs to be done with focus and intent. For this reason it was decided that so many untrained people would not be able to keep their concentration on the purpose. It was decided to put off the dance until another year, giving time for practices to be held to ensure that the weaving would go smoothly. (The jumping over the Beltane fire was done, however.)

This decision still did not answer the question of what energy was behind the May pole, and if not actuated by the pole dance how else could it be expressed? The group chose to do other activities which would express the essence of Beltane in different ways, but it was not an easy process and I have no hard-and-fast rules on how to proceed. The best I can offer when deciding what to plan for your seasonal events is to be open to inner guidance and trust that you will be guided by the Spirit to do what is right for the community at that time.

Below are listed two outlines of seasonal rituals that I have conducted in the past. The first is from a four-day Samhain celebration, and the second is from an Imbolc festival that lasted two and a half days. My purpose here is not to lay out a blueprint to be blindly copied, but more to offer suggestions from which to begin planning your own ceremonial events.

Books that offer guided visualizations or other process work, as well as books that describe seasonal rites, can be consulted for more ideas. The outlines below show nothing but a structure that may be followed, not the content of a ritual itself. There are endless possibilities that are available to groups willing to experiment.

OUTLINE OF A 4-DAY Samhain event

Note: this ceremony combines a space for seasonal teachings in the Celtic Tradition, but it also contains time for personal prayer and meditation. The organization of the clans and their duties will be discussed in more detail in Chapter Two. "Elders," here, means the facilitators of the event. Also, where the outline mentions "dancers," it means the participants in the ritual.

Wednesday evening.

Set up the altars and decorate and cleanse the site. (This could be done Thursday morning if the hall is not available the night before.)

Day One – Ritual begins: Thursday evening.

A. Participants arrive. After administrative details are taken care of, they visit the Altar dedicated specifically to the Spirits of the Place—outside the space set aside for the main event. Upon their return participants are cleansed and gather within the Sacred Circle itself inside the ceremonial hall. Once inside the sacred space participants should refrain from idle chatter with friends. Stay outside until you are ready to focus on the true reason you've come.

B. When it's time to begin, a potted small tree or large container of branches is brought into the hall by a group of the participants. While everyone sings, the tree is set into place within the centre of the Circle. Warned ahead of time, participants may come forward one at a time to tie small ribbons on the tree and state their pledges for the dance. Next the Circle is cast, with the four clan leaders calling in the Guardians of the Directions and other elders invoking the Goddess and the God.

C. The body of work for the first evening is the opening Council. This talking-stick circle is a very structured affair. While the stick is being passed, only the person holding it has the right to speak. Dancers are asked specific questions, such as "Who are you? What do you do in the world? What do you

hope to get from this experience, and what are you willing to give in return?"
As the stick is passed, the questions are repeated by each member so that we
stay on track. With between twenty and fifty people to speak, a time limit of
three minutes per person is imposed. Someone keeps time with a stop watch
and rings a little bell when the time for each speaker is up.

D. After the stick has completed the circle, the elders give general
information about the event and tell some teaching stories if there is time.

E. The evening ends with some drumming practice and a personal short
visit with the elders for people wishing to draw a Tarot card, rune or other
divination system and receive personal guidance for their dance over the next
few days.

F. The ritual closes down for the night. For this night, people could either
sleep on the site or go home, as they choose.

Day Two: Friday morning.

A. Short leaders' meeting and clan time.

B. The Circle is cast. Opening exercises. The Salmon clan leader teaches
the dance steps to the yang and yin outer circles. (The yang and yin circles are
explained in detail later.)

Morning Break.

C. Elders give some of the teachings connected to the rite.

Lunch.

Friday afternoon:

D. After lunch, clans separate to plan a five-minute opening each clan will
present this evening to honor their directions and open the Dance for the
night.

E. If there is time, a drumming practice can happen, and then quiet time
until the evening event begins. Participants may wish to visit the Altar to the
Place again or meditate. Idle chatter is discouraged during this time. This isn't
free time, it is part of ceremony set aside for inner reflection and preparation.
To prepare for the evening, everyone is also expected to adorn themselves in
their best ceremonial regalia and paint.

Friday evening: Feast of the Dead

F. This feast is to honor our ancestors. To do this, a plate is prepared with
a little of everything on the table. Later it will be placed outside on the Altar

of the Place for the rest of the night. After the ancestors have been honored, everyone else is fed.

G. After the feast, the Dance begins with a grand procession into the ceremonial space. When all is ready, the Circle is cast by the four clans presenting their invocations to the spirits of the four directions prepared during the afternoon. The elders invoke the Gods in the center of the ceremonial space.

H. First presentation is the give-away ceremony (explained later).

I. For this first night, participants are allowed to dance in the yang and yin rings only. The Dance continues until it seems appropriate to close down for the night. After that, a ban of silence should be enforced until the next morning. Not all the dancers attending this larger event have spent several weeks in meditation and preparation like the core group. For this reason it is important to build into the structure of the ceremony itself the time the dancers will require to do the inner work needed to benefit from the next night's longer event. Once the circle is cast and the rite begins, only necessary talking in low tones should be permitted throughout the event. Dragon clan members should see that this is carried out. (And that includes the smokers clustered in the parking lot if they can be heard by other dancers inside the sacred circle.)

J. Dancers are expected to stay within the ceremonial Circle by bringing in bedding and sleeping on the dance ground for the rest of the night. Keeping people on site helps maintain and build spiritual energy.

Day Three: Saturday morning.

A. Short leaders' meeting and clan time after breakfast.

B. The Circle is renewed. Opening exercises and more dance practice.

Break.

C. A walking meditation in which members walk in figure-eight movements around the paths of the inner circle, asking themselves, "At the ritual tonight, what part of me do I want to let go of – who will die?" "Who will be reborn from this experience?" (See the diagram of the walking meditation (Figure 1) at the end of this chapter.)

Lunch.

Saturday afternoon:

D. A teaching about drumming and chanting. Dancers are taught how to use their voices in wordless chants that can be used in the ceremony that night.

A practice if there is time or another talking stick circle within each clan can happen.

Short Break:

E. Dancers assemble to sit quietly and hear a guided visualization/story that depicts a seasonally appropriate teaching, such as the telling of the descent of the Goddess Inanna into the Underworld. Participants with no other duties after that can have smaller talking stick circles or nap until dinner.

During the late afternoon while a meal is being prepared and the hall decorated for the Underworld drama, those who have been "called spiritually" to be in the sacred drama enacted that night will need time to discuss their part and quietly meditate as they invoke the divine power they will channel.

Dinner:

F. After a light meal eaten with their clans, dancers put on simple white robes or loose clothing and file out of the hall to another room or area, to wait quietly blindfolded for Lord or Lady Death to come and claim them. (If time is an issue, instead of taking everyone individually, they can be brought to the gate of the underworld by clans.)

G. Death's servant brings the blindfolded dancers to the gate of the Underworld (the entrance to the main hall). They are asked to leave behind a piece of jewelry or other meaningful personal token, to symbolize letting go of their attachment to the living world.

To also symbolize the seriousness of this moment the gate-keeper may hold, an object like a butter knife to the dancer's neck while asking the question, "Who dies?" (The question refers to unwanted aspects of the self, and the answer is expected to be something like "He who is always lonely" or "She who creates destructive relationships.") If a participant does not have an answer, he or she is returned to the waiting area to think, until an answer comes.

Once inside, each dancer is blessed with ashes by another servant of the Underworld, then brought to stand or sit quietly, blindfolded in the dark hall, until all is ready for the next part. The purpose of this is not to learn how to find one's way without sight, but to try to imagine how it would feel to be dead. After a time a drum is sounded, the blindfolds are removed, and the Ruler of the Underworld speaks to the assembled dancers, asking them why they have come, and who of their ancestors do they wish to call upon to be near them this night. The Ruler will also ask if the dancers wish a gift of the Darkness, or help with some personal issue the dancer is working on. When all is ready, the evening Dance will begin.

H. The Ruler of the Underworld casts the Circle and invites the Dancers within the sacred space. (Because we are drawing upon Underworld "Earth energy," I usually cast this Circle counter-clockwise, and close the Circle in a clockwise direction when dancers emerge from the Underworld.)

I. The Dance in the Halls of the Underworld begins. For the first few hours, dancers stay on the outer rings as they did the night before. Later, as the night progresses and the dancers deepen into a light trance, the inner circle is opened and dancers may enter to express their own Dance as they see fit. Some of the Salmon clan members take turns watching over the inner circle to see that no one bumps into another or gets into trouble with their Dance.

J. Near dawn, the Dance winds to a close. A fire is lit in a cauldron, and dancers come forward to place an offering in the flames and say goodbye to the ancestors who have been with them throughout the night.

K. The Circle is opened (clockwise) and the dancers file out of the Underworld in a spiral procession. At the gate to the Underworld they are asked the question, "Who is conceived this night?" (If a Beltane ritual is planned as well for the same participants, they will revisit the Underworld at that time, and the Ruler will ask them, "Who has been born with the Spring?") They are now brushed with cedar bows and blessed with water, corn-meal or another sacred herb. After the blessing dancers will walk outside for morning prayers and chants. Dancers then return to the hall.

A note here about sleep. When I learned from Elizabeth she always allowed participants to take a short hour or hour and a half nap at this point. You may wish to do that, because most modern participants aren't used to going without sleep for this long. However, I have been taught by my Indigenous Elders that it's better to remain awake until your next sleeping cycle the following evening.

I personally agree with this. I've found that a nap after being up all night in sacred ceremony only dulls my wits and makes me feel even more tired after the brief nap. This to some extent is a personal choice, and the more you participate in sacred ceremonies lasting for longer periods the easier it will become. Part of the newcomer's reluctance to stay up for such a long time is mental rather than just physical.

Day Four: Sunday morning.

Breakfast.

A. After the meal is the closing Council. Five minutes is now allotted to each participant, so this will take some time. As with the opening Council, the dancers are asked specific questions, such as, "What were the highlights of the ritual for you? What did you have trouble with during the ceremony? What will you take away with you from this experience?"

B. After the Council, the Circle is opened and dancers bid farewell to the spirits of the Dance and of the site.

C. Don't everybody rush off while the clan leaders take down and pack their shrines. The East and South clans organize and proceed with clean-up, with other clans' help if possible.

This concludes the outline of this particular rite. All this should be laid out in detail during the planning phase of the process. At the actual event, things may have to be shifted around a little for time considerations, but it's better to over-plan than to have a lot of empty time that will let the energy be drained away.

⊗

OUTLINE OF A 2½-DAY Imbolg event

Friday evening.

A. We assemble at 6:00 (please be prompt) for registration.

B. Opening Council begins at 7:00. After an opening prayer and simple Circle casting, we have an outline of the event, some ceremonial teachings and a talking-stick circle (with time limits per person). If time permits, some drumming and chanting. Break for the night.

Saturday morning.

A. Short leaders' meeting and clan time. Opening prayer and casting of the Circle. Questions. The teaching of the steps to the outer (yang and yin) lines of the Dance circle, also drumming practice.

Break.

B. The teachings of the season, asking the question "To what do you dedicate your Dance?"

Lunch.

Saturday afternoon.

C. The walking meditation of the Creator-Destroyer, in which members walk in figure-eight movements around the paths of the inner circle, asking themselves, "What am I creating in my life?" "What am I destroying?" (See the diagram of the walking meditation (Figure 1) at the end of this chapter.)

D. Quiet time and or guided visualization.

Break.

E. After this, silence is asked for, to give dancers time to rest and to look within for spiritual guidance and growth. (It is also a good idea for newcomers to try to catch a nap; it will be a long night.)

Saturday evening.

Feast.

F. When all is ready, the dancers are dressed and painted, and food is prepared, we begin with a feast.

G. After the feast comes the Give-away.

The Long Dance:

H. We begin by casting the Circle and inviting the Goddess and God to join us.

I. The Dance begins. For the first few hours, all dancers stay on the two outer circles of the Dance. Later, as we deepen into the trance experience, the inner circle is opened for the personal Dance. Near dawn we return to the yin and yang lines.

J. The Dance ends with a blessing and the closing of the Circle.

Sunday morning.

A. Dawn prayers and chants at the Altar to the Place.

Breakfast

B. The closing Council.

C. Clean-up.

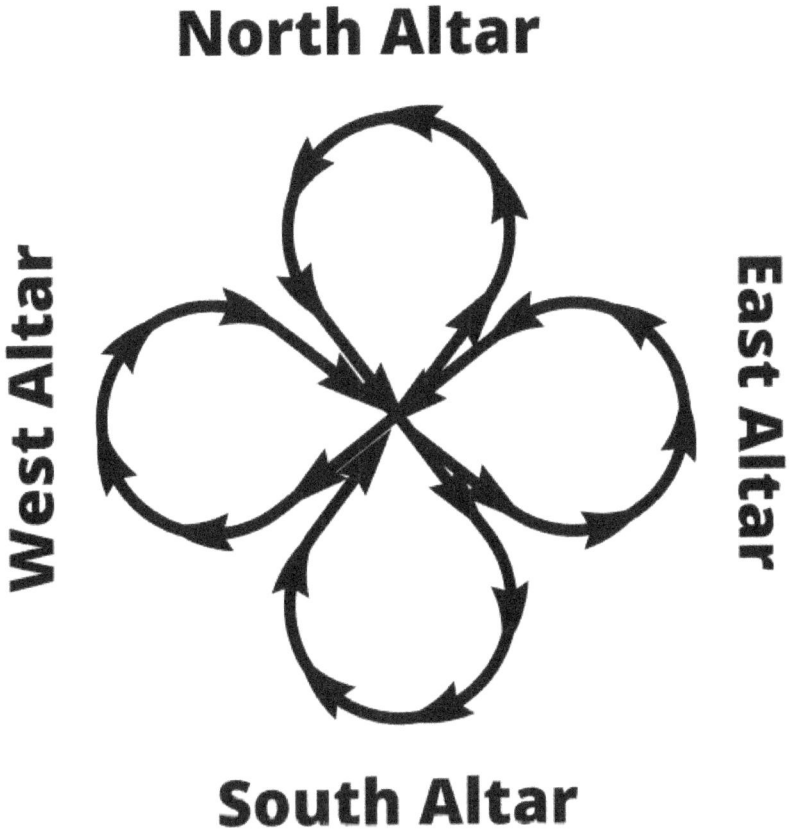

North Altar

West Altar

East Altar

South Altar

Figure 1: Walking Meditation

A double-figure-8 walking meditation is designed to allow participants in a ritual to concentrate upon a pair of questions. The group splits into two subgroups. One subgroup walks the North-South figure 8 and concentrates upon the first question, while the other subgroup walks the East-West figure 8 and concentrates on the second question. Midway in the meditation, they switch places, so everyone walks both figure 8's and consider both questions.

FINANCING EVENTS

I have just realized that nowhere yet have I talked about financing these events. Well, no better time than now. Traditionally, money was not supposed to enter into the matter of planning and performing a ceremony. Goods and services were exchanged instead. However, that doesn't always work today. I don't agree that these rituals should be big profit-making events, because I believe in the idea of service to the community, but if there is to be a community ritual, then the community must support it. That usually means money must be raised for hall rental, food, and other expenses. The best way I've found to do this is to figure out all the possible expenses and divide it up by the number of participants you hope to have attend.

Your group may run up against a situation in which there are people in your community who may wish to attend but may not have the money at that time to do so. I know of two ways to work with that problem that I can offer as suggestions for how to handle money issues. This whole subject is not easy. I try to always keep in mind that we are in a time of transition, in which our ceremonies are part workshop, in the modern sense, and part traditional rite. There is no way for most of us to get around that fact.

Money is needed for expenses, and, if that is explained to people, with an estimate of how much is needed from each person, and then donations are asked for, often that is enough. The other way is to set a firm price based on your expenses and tell people that a ceremony is an energy exchange; in order to get something out of it, you need to be willing to give something in return. If you don't have the money right now, then make a spiritual commitment to pay what you can now and the rest whenever you can. The spirits will know if you don't keep your word, and will act accordingly.

This is risky for the organizers, and brings up all kinds of issues around trust, but it usually works. For the type of ceremonial process that I teach, work trades aren't appropriate, because everyone has tasks to do during the event and afterwards. That is part of the learning process of the ceremony itself, so it is better to get clear around money and stick to the core group's decision.

I believe the ideal number of participants is no less than twenty, because it is hard to raise enough group energy to carry through the whole process with fewer people, and no more than fifty, because the group is then too large and impersonal to achieve good results with more than that. This is my experience, but it will be up to your group to decide what will work best for your particular event.

I said that I recommend no more than fifty active participants in a ritual. This may seem quite a small number, especially to those who have attended Native or other cultural events where hundreds of people take part. If you look at those ceremonies more closely, however, you will usually find that most attendees take on the role of a witness to the rite, rather than an initiate to the deeper mysteries. The witness is an important role, and helps strengthen community bonding, reaffirming connections and unity among different factions in the society.

For most of us twenty to fifty participants is a workable number. Children, spouses, or other interested persons can be encouraged to attend portions of a long ceremony as witnesses, and the role of witness is also useful for people nervous about attending a long ritual for the first time, but always separate the deeper mysteries from the uninitiated. For example, in a Samhain event centering on a descent into the Underworld, witnesses must not enter the Underworld or meet the Lord or Lady Death.

Another point that usually comes up with new participants is the question of whether they can come late to the event. In general, I would say no, but there have been times when I have had to break that rule. Usually if there are sacred teachings involved that dancers will need to participate fully in the ceremony it just doesn't work for these dancers to come in late. Not only have they missed vital teachings, they have also missed a chance to fully mesh their energies with other dancers and the ceremony itself.

While on the other hand, if the rite isn't too deep and more for celebration and fun, the latecomer can intermesh quite well. There is a balance here between the need for commitment and discipline on the one hand, with the need to give as many people as possible the chance to experience the deeper aspects of ceremony.

In the past, I have been criticized by some elders for being too easy on newcomers. I recognize that that is a problem, but I have chosen to be easy and reach a larger group of people, rather than be more disciplined and reach far fewer. As it is, many inexperienced dancers consider me frighteningly strict. To paraphrase: How do you know if you like ice cream if you never had a chance to taste it? Some may decide ice cream is not for them, while others may decide they like it so much they want to help make it, and they might never have discovered they liked it at all if they had not been given a chance to taste it.

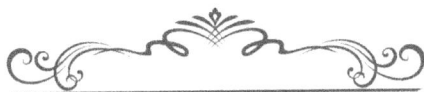

Chapter 2

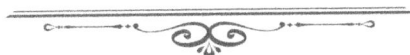

Step 2:
The Preparation of a Ceremony

In the previous chapter, on planning, I talked about the structure of long ceremonies and when to perform them, but not a lot was said about the organization or about how things get done. In this next step, let's begin with some suggestions on how to accomplish the many tasks that need to be done to perform an elaborate ritual. It is important, I believe, to divide the work as evenly as possible, so that no one person suffers from burn-out, either before, during, or after the rite.

FORMING THE CORE GROUP

It goes without saying that a core group of committed members will need to meet together regularly to create the final rite. Any way your group chooses to divide up the work will be the right way for that time, but I would like to suggest creating a system of four clans to which every participant at the ceremony will belong. The clan system, for me, is connected to each of the four cardinal directions and the four elements, and each clan has certain responsibilities that are connected with its element. Below are listed the clans that I use. If they are in harmony with the ritual system that you have created, please use them. If not, feel free to adapt them as you choose.

A further note here about the clan system: everyone attending the ceremony will need to join one of the four clans created for the rite when they show up on the first day of the event. Not everyone who is called to participate need spend the two or three month preparation beforehand like the clan elders and organizers. However, because each clan has specific duties throughout the ceremony everyone present needs to join one of the four clans. Unless you have decided to include the role of the witness in your rite, but if that is the case then the people choosing to witness only witness. They can't start participating as dancers part way through the ritual, (if they feel the vibe).

How the newcomers choose their clan affiliation can be a tricky problem, because you want the group to be equally divided among the clans. Since each clan has responsibilities you can't have one clan with three people and another with fifteen just because that's what the participants think they have an affinity for one clan over another. You will have to decide how to divide the participants in some way, so I offer this suggestion.

With new arrivals on the first night I have sometimes asked the newcomers to count off numbers 1 to 4 around the circle. Then all the number one join the air clan, all the number twos join the fire clan and so on... there is room for exceptions here if a new person has expertise in something needed by a particular clan, but sometimes it's also good to go with the challenge of doing something new and outside your comfort zone.

The Deer Clan – direction: North – element: Earth

Spiritually, this clan identifies with Earth. Its clan elder is responsible for gathering together items for, and erecting, the North altar at the festival site. On a mundane level, Earth honors our physical reality, so all the practical details like registration (in whatever form this takes for you), payment, and food preparation belong to the Deer People. The qualities of this clan are nurturing, self-sacrifice, and abundance. This doesn't mean that the North Clan has to prepare all the food or do all the work; it merely means that they organize things so that the work gets done. During the event itself, they set out nutritious snacks and organize meals. After the event is over, their work is mostly finished; others will be responsible for clean-up.

The Loon or Wild Goose Clan – direction: East – element: Air

Spiritually, this clan identifies with Air. The clan elder is responsible for gathering what is necessary to set up the East altar. One of the main qualities of Air is sound and communication, so these Bird Clan people would be in charge of things like social media advertising, mail-outs, phone calls and other similar duties. During the event, this clan's primary function is to maintain the sound field – i.e., drumming and chanting. This does not mean that members of other clans can't join in drumming or chanting; it merely means that the East Clan is responsible for the music. This is an important function, because the drum is the heartbeat of the Dance, and its use can determine the success or failure of a rite. After the ritual is over, the East Clan members stick around to help clean up the space – blowing away all traces of our passing, like the wind.

The Dragon Clan – direction: South – element: Fire

Spiritually, this clan identifies with Fire. Its clan elder sets up the South altar. The Dragon People's main function (and it's a hard one) is security and overseeing the energy levels of the Dance. The Dragons are our outer ring of protection; they see that unwelcome people do not invade the energy of the rite. (For example, if the Fire Marshall comes by to see that everything is safe, the Dragon Clan elder must speak to him.) It is the responsibility of the Dragons to enforce rules of silence when that is called for. They also maintain the energy of the Dance, which may mean getting out on the Dance floor at three o'clock in the morning with energetic dancing to get everybody moving again. This clan's security duties may sound harsh, but bear in mind that their responsibility is to maintain the energy of the event, and anything that either threatens the ritual or draws energy away from it is their rightful concern. After the ceremony, they help with clean-up (transforming the hall back to its normal state). Beforehand, their duties are more free-floating. They can help where needed. In some groups, they help prepare the ceremonial site or store and protect the altar items until they are needed again.

The Orca or Salmon Clan – direction: West – element: Water

This clan's spiritual element (as you can guess) is Water, and their clan elder sets up the West altar. Their functions are related to the Water element, but are somewhat diverse. The Orca Clan teaches the dances and their steps to the members of the other clans, and when the inner circle is opened for the trance dancing, they take turns watching to make sure no one gets into trouble by going "too deep" into their own processes. On a more mundane level, the West Clan makes sure our watery refreshments are always overflowing during the event. (They can also do dishes, if the Deer Clan lets them in the kitchen.)

Before the event, their tasks centre around movement—picking up out-of-town people, shopping for supplies, getting people, firewood, or goods from place to place, etc. Members of this clan have also been used as mediators and advisors when group conflicts occur or inner work needs to be done.

The clan system, as I have outlined it here, is an attempt to recreate for modern people a workable method of organization that is similar to that used by traditional cultures around the world. At present, it is still rather loosely structured, with lots of room for individual community experimentation. The advantage I feel that the clans have over a system where different people in the core group are assigned tasks at random is that, with the clan system, over time, a spiritual connection can be added to the work.

This is what is missing today, but was so much a part of most traditional systems – the linking of the physical and spiritual aspects of ceremony. In our modern era, we all too often compartmentalize things and forget about their blending. With the clans, there are layer upon layer of meanings that can be drawn from the tasks associated with the clan office. Discovering the deeper spiritual connections associated with an element will take time and some inner work and meditation. For most of us who don't have a council of elders from which to draw wisdom, it will mean exploring within ourselves to find the answers.

The term "clan elder" may seem a little presumptuous at first (especially since I said earlier that I don't consider anyone under sixty to be an elder), but a word is needed to recognize that someone is responsible for both the spiritual and physical duties of the clan. "Clan leader" or "clan mother or father" can be used instead, if your group prefers it. Ideally, this person (or persons) should be self-chosen, by feeling a spiritual call from the sacred energy of one element to serve it. The clan elder should be a person who has expertise with some aspects of the work that is associated with that clan. I'm speaking ideally, of course. In reality, that expertise takes time to develop, so no one with the necessary experience may be available for the first few rituals your group performs.

For some groups, no matter how the duties are delegated, the clan system won't work. For them, the tasks simply need to be divided among group members until the group as a whole has had more time and experience in working together.

For other groups, the physical and spiritual duties of the clan will work best if given to more than one person to take charge of. Thus, clan elders may have their own helpers, or there might be two or three elders in a clan.

Whatever modifications of the clans you may choose to adopt, I would suggest keeping the same people in place for more than one ceremony. This will give the clan leaders time to deepen their spiritual awareness of the elements they serve, as well as time to perfect the organization of the physical tasks to be done. I would suggest not changing to another element for at least a year's cycle, to begin with.

Clan elders may wish to keep a clan book or diary in which their spiritual insights are recorded and clan duties are clearly stated. These books eventually become a history of a community's spiritual growth, and are an invaluable resource when it comes time to pass on the leadership of a clan to another person.

To prevent small misunderstandings from growing into major rifts in the community, it is important to establish very clear boundaries of who does what within the clan itself, and between clans within the ceremony as a whole. It is important to work out as much as possible before the ceremony. During the ceremony it is also a good idea to schedule both clan time (when the whole clan meets) and clan elder time (when the elders meet together in the core group), so that everyone knows what is going on. This will help prevent problems that may crop up later.

As someone once described it to me, a ceremony is like a theatre production; there is the director who has over-all responsibility to see that the show goes on, and then there are all the others who have areas of responsibility and expertise who are in charge of various duties that, when put all together, make up the whole show. So, with that analogy in mind, there are elders who are responsible for the whole of the ceremony, and clan leaders who are responsible for the various parts.

It stands to reason that the clan elders are solely in charge of their areas of expertise. Just as make-up shouldn't tell the sound-man how to do his job in the theatre, so each clan needs to respect the boundaries of the others' responsibilities. These are all boundary issues, and a part of the group process that must be worked out if the ceremonial system is to grow and prosper over time.

As I envision it, eventually the clans will grow stable and strong enough so that each clan in a community can sponsor one of the seasonal rites. I would also envision a system in which each person has a home clan of affinity, then after gaining some wisdom in that clan they go on to be apprentices in each of the other clans, eventually returning to their home clans as more balanced people.

I digress. Getting back to the dance, I would also suggest creating an information sheet for new members to tell them about the clans and their roles, as well as giving general information about the ceremony itself. There is so much to learn and discuss that it is hard to cover it all in the short time allotted for the rite itself. The sheets are one way to handle this dilemma. They also help participants decide which clan they want to join.

I have mentioned before that people are called by the ceremony itself to participate in the event. The same holds true in the beginning stages as well. A person must feel a call and want to serve. It will only lead to trouble and hard feelings if this is not respected.

The great temptation here is to want to appoint a friend because you just know that person would be right for the job. Though the motivation may be good, in the end this type of appointment usually backfires. If people are ready, they will volunteer; until then, it is best to carry on as well as you can. (Of course, you can ask people if they want to help prepare for an event; otherwise, they may not know the opportunity is there. "We're getting together a core group to create a 4-day Beltane ritual. Do you want to be part of it?")

Ideally, again, I would see the core group that plans and prepares for the ceremony as consisting of at least the four clan leaders and one or two assistants. There should also be one or more wise elders whose duty it is to oversee and channel power to the ceremony as a whole. In the European Pagan tradition, these elders would represent the Goddess and God, just as the clan elders represent the power of the four elements.

At first, there may not be so many willing to commit to the long preparations needed, so compromises will have to be made. For the first Long Dance I did after studying with my teacher Elizabeth, I tended to almost everything myself, even catering the food. I did this because I felt very strongly that I was called to give the experience of this type of ceremony to my home community. At the time, it did not feel like a burden or a lot of work. One task flowed into the next without effort. My mind was so focused on the work that it was almost like being in meditation for two months.

During this time, I still had a family to take care of, so I couldn't retreat from the everyday world to concentrate only on the ceremony. How I managed I think was more a question of organization and putting to better use, those hours of dead time that we all have and don't make use of, rather than suddenly acquiring super-powers.

It is not my place to be judgmental about what others do. I would only say that we have a choice, and each of us decides what our interests are and how we choose to use our time. To practice community ceremonials may only mean looking beyond a mind-set that causes limitations to one that is more open to possibilities you may not have considered. Also, it is a good idea to think of it as an honor to be called to serve an element, rather than "Oh, God, I've got to do all this work."

GROUP SPIRITUAL PREPARATION

When the organizational details have been decided upon, the preparation step itself begins. As I have stated before, in many cultures, preparation for a seasonal ceremony takes months of hard work. I believe very strongly that it is time to re-establish that kind of devotion and commitment in our modern Pagan communities. There are no short-cuts to magical power and enlightenment, there just aren't. If you are in harmony with what you are doing, it will seem like a joy, not a burden, to do the work needed for the ritual. If you are not in harmony with what you are doing, it is best not to do it at all. (Also, it is very true that "many hands make light work." Doing the work together with the other members of the core group is likely to be much easier than doing the same amount of work alone.)

I like to take at least two to three months to prepare for a long ritual event. When you make a time commitment each day to focus some of your mental and physical energy on the upcoming ceremony, a depth of feeling and power is yours that can never be there in any other way.

In all our Pagan sacred rites, one or more human agents must act as channels for the divine energies. To do this properly takes discipline and training. If there are no trained people present at a rite, the Gods may choose someone who is sensitive or vulnerable through whom to manifest their power, or the energies may remain a chaotic force with no guidance within the ritual. In either case, the results can be upsetting and dangerous.

I am not talking about zombie-like possession here, when I speak of channeling the Divine. I am merely referring to the light trance-channeling that most good spiritual healers use all the time. This is the state in which healers feel energized and guided to do what is necessary for the task at hand. If you know how to channel properly, you can act as a conduit for spiritual energies, allowing the power to flow through you without draining you.

If I feel drained or exhausted after a healing session or a ritual, I know I've done something wrong. I've invested too much of myself in the work, and not enough of the divine force has been able to get through my personal blocks. For this reason, it is necessary for the core group, and anyone else wishing to make a personal commitment, to meet regularly to do the inner work that will enable them to channel the divine power properly.

I ask clan leaders and other core participants to meet at least twice a month—and weekly is better—for two or three months prior to the ceremony to do some of this inner work together. At these meetings, the group discusses practical problems that may arise, as well as doing exercises to deepen their understanding of the season and the theme of the coming festival.

I encourage people to keep a daily diary of their dreams and meditational insights. I also ask that they create their robes of office and pull together the ritual tools and items to be used in the decoration of the shrines (if they are the keepers of those shrines). For the Underworld ceremony outlined in Chapter One, there was the sacred theatre of the Underworld to prepare for as well. Other seasonal rites will have other needs.

Some people may be afraid of such a commitment, but it is not an overwhelming task. Like the idea of dancing all night, it may seem impossible at first, but as you go along the energy builds and you find it quite easy, or at least not as hard as you had expected. Meeting regularly means that you are able to draw on group support and energy for your own personal work as well.

At this point, the question would probably arise of what kind of exercises or devotions need to be done by the group and by persons wishing to experience this deeper commitment. I am reluctant to lay out an outline, for fear it will be followed too rigidly, since trusting your intuitions is part of the process. I can, however, offer some ideas and suggestions on how to proceed.

First of all, your group may wish to decide whether to meet as a whole, or separately by clans (if you have a large core group) or do a little of both.

Some meetings will need to be dedicated to practical administrative details, such as food preparation or advertising costs. For other meetings, however, your purpose in coming together for that session will be to work on group process dedicated to achieving a spiritual bonding; in this case, it is important not to allow your gatherings to bog down in gossip sessions or too many details of preparation. Try to set aside separate times for those discussions.

Your first lesson in this process is the discipline of staying focused on the topic the group has agreed upon for a given session. If it is a spiritual exercise, stick to that. As in Eastern meditations where the initiate concentrates his mind on the breath, the focus on the topic of your meeting can be equally challenging, only in this case it is the group mind rather than the individual that is challenged.

If your group is planning a seasonal rite, then I would recommend spending some of your time together trying to understand and connect with the sacred forces that are present at those times. This can be done by talking to elders, by study and research, or through guided visualizations in which you experience the power that season has to offer. If you plan to meet by clans, your clan may wish to do similar exercises for its particular element as well.

For group ritual, the purpose of preparation is always to enhance the skills needed to enact your ceremony. Drumming, chanting, dancing, and regalia and mask making are skills that will deepen your ceremonial practice as well as fostering group oneness. Such things as drumming and song, and guided visualizations on agreed-upon topics, would be good beginnings for these twice-monthly sessions.

To achieve a type of group mind that will enhance ceremonial work requires that the group be able to work out any personal conflicts between the members. For true unity and telepathic communication to occur, a bond of trust must be established. This book cannot go into group processes in enough detail to give you directions and guidelines, but I know this process work must be done, and I would refer you to several good books in the bibliography that may be of assistance should problems arise. I recommend both Mendel's *The Leader as Martial Artist*, and Starhawk's *Truth or Dare* for this purpose.

For those who stick out the process, in time things will come together, and then your ritual will achieve previously-unimagined depths of meaning and power. I can't stress enough the importance of sticking through the process.

There is a lot of talk these days about going back to traditional values and forming community. Certainly most of us need to connect with others in a world that is fragmented and sterile, but there are no short-cuts and most people don't have the patience or the courage to work through all the conflicts needed to achieve lasting results.

I say "the conflicts needed to achieve lasting results," because it almost seems to be a natural law that conflicts will arise, and it's pointless to hope they won't; you've just got to deal with them. Too many groups break up as soon as there is a disagreement, and never handle it. We're really good at working alone, but not together; our whole society stresses competition rather than co-operation. This is why we find it so hard to stay together in the groups we form. It is the challenge of our time, to learn to work together in groups.

There are two main ways that I can see to proceed in forming a ritual group. One would be to create a very intimate group that shares everything, and whose members work, live, or socialize together. There is, however, another way, wherein people come together to create and perform ritual, but do not choose to use the group for emotional sustenance, and members have other interests and support systems outside the group context.

In working together, personal conflicts and intimate issues are bound to arise, but in this second kind of group they do not become such a focus of group energies as in the first kind. Most traditional spiritual societies that I know of, operate closer to the second model, while most of the modern New Age spiritual circles tend to seek the total involvement of the first. In older, more established cultures, family ties take care of many of the functions that modern people expect from their group connections. This dependence on the group is okay in theory, but in practice may put added strains on group members wishing to come together only to do ritual. It will be up to the group as a whole to determine how involved with each other they wish to be.

INDIVIDUAL SPIRITUAL Preparation

Along with group preparations, individuals may wish to do some personal work. This, to me, can take the form of daily meditations, keeping a diary, or deciding upon a personal pledge. A personal pledge is a commitment made by someone asking for guidance from the spirit realm. Such pledges are a form of self-sacrifice. It is a type of energy exchange, and the laws of the universe say that if you want to get something you've got to be willing to give something in return.

This may sound confusing or vague, so let me give some examples. If I wish to find a house or land to buy and am not having any luck finding just the right place by conventional means, I may wish to do magic to help things along. Suppose I also know that a big ceremony is coming up in two months. I make a pledge to be at that ceremony and that between now and then I will do inner work, and I agree to give up something I enjoy or that means a lot to me. *Means a lot to me*, this is important, and I can't stress this strongly enough. Your gift must have equal value spiritually as the gift you are asking for in return. What I give up is the pledge I make in exchange for help in getting what I want, and there can be no cheating.

Pledges may be made to ask for tangible things like a house or a new job, or they may be about emotional issues like controlling an addiction or working through problems in a relationship. Pledges can also be made to benefit others (with their permission), or for the well-being of the planet.

I remember years ago seeing the movie *Colors*, at my teenage boys' insistence. This movie is about drugs and violence in the Los Angeles ghetto communities. It had a deep effect on me. After leaving the theatre that night, I couldn't go home for two hours or more; I just walked about with tears streaming down my face. Living in the bush and rural areas of Canada, as I had been for a number of years, my family and I had been insulated from the urban reality many young people face. I guess having brown-skinned teenage boys of my own made the plight of children in the ghetto doubly real for me.

Not long after this, we had a summer ceremonial, and when the ribbons were put on the tree I dedicated the sacrifice of my dance to the children of the cities, so that, if they chose to accept its gift of power, my sacrifice could make their lives a little easier. I call my dance a "sacrifice" because great strength and energy are needed to endure a long ritual, and it's not always easy or pleasant. This means, however, that equally great power is available to be given away for any purpose I may choose.

For each of us, personal commitments and devotions are very individual. No one can give rules for another; you must do what is right for you, but I will offer some words of caution about how you choose what you are willing to give in an energy exchange.

-There are no bargains or fast deals; what you give is what you get.

-If you are asking for something important, you must be willing to offer something equally important in return.

The relative weight of your request and your pledge is not always as easy to decide as it may appear. A young girl I counselled once told me she had been fasting on juice and water for twenty days, as a pledge to help a political cause she was involved with. This might seem like a great spiritual gift, but the woman was a borderline anorexic. Fasting came easy to her; in fact, it was one of her problems.

I suggested that a greater gift to herself and her spirit guides would be to gain twenty pounds, and to feel good about herself as she did it. This was an enormously harder pledge for her, and so would have much more meaning for an energy exchange than the fasting she chose to do.

Many religious philosophies stress sacrifice far more than my own beliefs do. For me, a balance between self-love and self-sacrifice is necessary for the harmony of all life. For this reason I suggest caution when making pledges in exchange for spiritual guidance.

One last word – it is important that, if you do make a spiritual commitment, you pledge only as much as you can do. Your word is your bond, and something sworn to within the sacred Circle carries far more weight than words said in the mundane world.

What happens if you don't keep your pledges? It's not that God (or Goddess) comes down and hits you over the head with a club for breaking your promises, but, in magic words are concrete things, with power in themselves. So when you break your word and don't keep your commitments, you are saying, to yourself and to the Universe, that you can't be trusted. Your self-esteem and credibility will suffer, and there's no point in doing ritual if you don't believe in what you're doing and take it seriously.

For this reason, it is important to make a spiritual pledge only when you feel ready to make a commitment to the task. No matter what others think or are doing, only do what is right for you at that time.

PHYSICAL PREPARATION

A short word about the physical preparations for a ritual, i.e. regalia, masks, and other tools. Money is not the important issue here. Using things you find or make, or buy from second-hand stores, is fine. Whatever you use, the thing to remember here is to cleanse the items and dedicate them to a ritual use. If you want these objects to stay strong and to store up energy from one event to another, they must be kept separate and only worn or used during ritual occasions. These physical symbols are important—they are concrete manifestations of our spiritual reality, and so should be treated with respect.

Many people argue that "real" spirituality doesn't need all this show. In a sense they are right. For your personal devotions, you may or may not wish to don ritual gear and perform long rites. A simple meditation may be enough. For group rites, however, I believe it is essential to use a variety of ritual props and regalia. All over the world, group rites are celebrated with a certain amount of pageantry, for a very good reason. All these masks, costumes, and power objects help the members of a group to focus on using similar mental imagery. The special robes and tools also send a message to our unconscious that this is sacred space, and that the rules of the everyday world no longer apply.

During the preparation stage, I find that making ritual gear is a meditation that helps me concentrate my energies on the coming festival. In order to focus on the things you are creating, it is important to do them with conscious intent. What that means, in practical terms, is not to sit down and sew regalia, for example, while watching *Star Trek*. If you watch TV shows or other forms of entertainment that distract part of your awareness while making your gear, the play of emotion that you experience from the external source will be reflected in the work that you produce, and your ritual robes will contain emotions and energies that may not be appropriate for their intended use. Listen to music, or chant, or in some way keep your energies focused on your spiritual task, so that the object you are creating will be a thing of power.

One further point: physical objects can take on and store power, or house spirits of their own. If you wish to invite and keep power within your tools, they must be treated with respect and not left out or displayed in your living room for idle hands to touch or break. Be careful of who, and what energies, your sacred things are exposed to. In general, ritual objects need to be cleansed and empowered, and shown honor. Treat them as more than just physical things, and let them get to know you.

And, every once in a while, offer them something such as food or drink (symbolically) to show your thankfulness and respect. If you've done your preparations right and a spirit is invested in a mask or a tool, you can talk to it and it will give you its name and tell you what it needs. You can offer food and drink to a mask, for instance, by placing the food before the mask and rubbing a little on its mouth—let the spirit tell you what it wants.

I would not offer food to a knife or a crystal; other forms of nurturing would be more appropriate. Depending on the physical composition of a tool, you can let it get to know you by holding it in your hands, covering it with your body's fluids, rubbing it with sacred oils, painting with ocher, smudging it with incense, or simply carrying it about with you – but always keeping the object at least in the back of your mind, even while you do other things. You, also, must get to know the object. Consider it as both an energy exchange and a partnership, where you and the tool or mask work together to achieve your joint ritual goals.

Since I do a lot of group rituals, I usually have two sets of ritual items – the personal ones that only I handle, and the group ones which are available for others to use. Many of my large crystals I feel have chosen me as their guardian because they wish to be used in group work in this way.

Traditional peoples around the world often spend a lifetime perfecting their ceremonial practices and going deeper in their understanding of ritual and its preparation. It's like the layers of an onion, always unfolding. You think you know it all, and then you find there's still more to learn. We as spiritual seekers need to make a commitment to that lifetime process of learning.

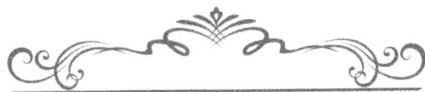

Chapter 3

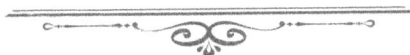

Step Three:
Creating Sacred Space

Site Selection

The first part of this step should have been decided upon during the planning phase (Step One), that is, where the ritual is to be held. Thinking about it logically, it would be reasonable to plan outdoor events for warm weather, and indoor rituals during the colder months. Weather patterns in the area in which the ceremony is to be held could make it advisable to have a back-up indoor facility in case of rain, even in warm weather.

(I'll never forget the summer solstice ritual when it poured rain the whole day, with nowhere to go and nothing to do but dance, soaking wet, in the rain, because the sponsor thought that it never rained at that time of year in her part of the country.) Remember, also, that it may be quite cold outside in the small hours of the morning, even in the middle of the summer, so if you do choose an outdoor site, make provision for people to get warm in some way.

Whatever site is chosen for an event, it should be as private as possible. It is important to seek isolation for the sake of personal trust and security. Drumming and chanting draw people like a magnet (evidence of their primal power for all human beings, of course). It is unsettling for everyone, and the energy fields of the rite will be affected, if uninformed outsiders are allowed to wander through the ceremonial grounds at will—especially if they are drunk or high. Therefore, it is advisable to choose the site carefully and have your security people (the Dragon Clan) alert to any interruption. An out-of-the-way community hall or deserted summer camp grounds are ideal places; their isolation offers privacy, and a minimum work load for the Dragon Clan.

Indoor events are easier to control than open fields, but the beauty of an open setting is a real plus for any rite. All too often, unfortunately, I have seen rituals planned with a mind to the beauty of the setting, but almost no care or thought given to the site itself. To run an outdoor event well takes a lot more work than meeting in a hall. For health and safety reasons, somebody's back hay field won't do. The ground needs to be cleaned and leveled, and tents or arbors need to be erected for shade and weather protection, as well as for easy access to food and water. You will be bringing in food, but you will find it much easier if fresh water is available on site, and you don't have to truck it in. (Fifty people need to drink an astonishing amount of water in four days.) Also, of course, some kind of bathroom/outhouse facilities must be available.

The best outdoor arrangements I've seen are put up by some Native reserves, where the dance area is outside, but the ground is carefully flattened or covered by a wooden floor and a shaded canopy covers part or all of the dance area. Ideally, groups that stay together for a while can create such a sanctuary, but, if not, give some real thought to the practicalities of an outdoor event, even in summer, before proceeding. You may find it easier to dance indoors, while holding other, shorter, parts of the ceremony outside.

There are several things to consider when planning for an outdoor event. First, because the dancers will be in light trance for part of the ritual, it is important to have a very level area, free of rocks and small holes where a dancer could trip and be injured. (Needless to say, all traces of horse or cow manure must be cleared away too!)

The second point to be cautious about in an open-air event is that there is a tendency to create an outdoor sacred space too large for the number of people gathered. The voice of a person giving announcements or sharing in talking circles doesn't always carry well outside. If the area is too large, it may become hard to hear from one side of the circle to the other. For best results, think small when working outside. The space should not exceed the dimensions of a moderate-sized hall; that way, everyone can see and hear, and the energy can stay focused where it needs to be, not out in the Great Beyond.

Thirdly, even if an event is scheduled to happen outside, consider a back-up place to go in case of poor weather. Trying to carry on with an event in the rain or cold can be uncomfortable and perhaps dangerous, as hours of cold, wet weather may cause hypothermia to develop with sensitive people. It's very hard to raise energy when everyone is wet and miserable.

For an indoor event, there are different considerations. For example, how much can your group afford to pay for hall rental? Are there kitchen facilities at the site? What are the acoustics like, and will you be allowed to make noise (such as drumming) after midnight? You may have to be creative; for example, if the hall is not isolated in itself, it should at least be isolatable. I once ran an event on the second floor of a factory in downtown Vancouver, but after the street doors were locked, it was in effect as isolated as a camp in the wilderness would have been.

SITE PREPARATION

In the example of the Samhain event outlined in Chapter One, a large rural community hall with a kitchen was chosen. The hall was transformed into a temple of sacred space the night before, and a guardian was left to sleep there while the rest of the work crew went home for a good rest after everything was prepared. It may not always be possible to set up the hall the night before an event, but it is important to allow lots of time for site preparation. It usually takes hours, and it's better if everyone has some time to rest and regroup before beginning the ritual itself.

A logical question to ask at this point is, why not wait until everyone arrives before setting up the site? For most New Age rituals, this is the way it is usually done. In these shorter rituals, there isn't a lot of prior spiritual preparation, so setting up the site at the time the ritual is to be performed replaces the longer preparation that I use, and helps focus the group on the rite about to be performed.

There is nothing wrong with this approach, but I prefer to prepare the site ahead of time, because, when you return to it at the beginning of the ritual itself, entering into a sacred temple, with the candles glowing and incense in the air, has a powerful effect on your unconscious, and you know this is serious stuff. It alerts your awareness to let go of everyday reality and be open to the realm of magic.

It is the clan elders' responsibility to take charge of the shrines and their decoration, but other participants can, and should, help out in other ways. There are a lot of things to do and the more people to help the better it will be. The exception to this is the altars themselves, where too many cooks can spoil the broth. The clan leader, and helper, if any, should be in a state of light trance while putting together the shrine. If they have been doing their daily meditations, they should have already been spiritually directed on how to arrange things.

The shrine should flow together very smoothly. It's funny, but by looking at the altars after they are set up, it is so apparent to me which clan elders have done their homework and which have not. I have watched people who have done the inner work ahead of time gain a deep resonance with the energy of their shrine. As they work, everything flows into place, then, later, the altar seems to vibrate with a special force. Other altars I look at are artistically well constructed, yet lifeless, because the creator of the altar either didn't do the inner work to prepare or was unable to channel the Sacred into a physical form.

Some participants in a rite may wish to bring items to be "charged" at a particular shrine. They must not put these things on the altar themselves, however; instead, they should give their objects to the clan leader of the desired element, who will decide where to put them in the arrangement of the altar. The clan leader may judge that an item does not "fit" the altar, i.e. that it is not suitable or appropriate for the design he or she has been guided to prepare. Such an item can still be charged with the energy of the element by being placed out of sight under the altar table. I would also suggest smudging or in some way cleansing these unknown items before they are added to any shrine.

Before even unpacking, the group that has come together to do set-up should gather together and have a group prayer and grounding meditation to help them center themselves and focus on the work at hand. The clan leaders, especially, need this time to become clear for their work. Also, it is wise to physically clean and symbolically cleanse the site, in order both to remove dirt and to change any negative energy patterns that may be hanging around, before you create any sacred shrine that could be affected by what has gone on before in that place. I'll explain more about how to go about the cleansing in the next step (Cleansing/Blessing).

No matter what layout you use, the four shrines to the directional guardians are large affairs set on tables or other platforms. They usually hold altar cloths, candles, crystals, and other items that reflect the elemental energy or the totem animal (Dragon, Orca, Deer, or Wild Goose, for example) connected with that direction. With outdoor shrines, I suggest a canopy be erected over the altar to protect it from the weather. If it is a permanent site, landscaping can be done to use Nature to display the symbols of the four elements.

The decoration of each shrine is left up to the clan leaders, but I would suggest that, if you plan to continue doing ritual as a group over time, you may acquire altar items that belong to the ceremony itself and are used over and over for each ritual event, and only for that purpose. Like other magical items, they will store power from one ceremony to the next.

I have four large boxes in my home that contain Long Dance gear, one for each altar. When the altars are put up each time, we use this material, with some additions from clan leaders or other participants. The shrines erected never look the same, but because the same objects are used, there is a special feeling about the items, and the shrines holding them, that comes from their repeated exposure to the Sacred.

CREATING THE INNER Circle:

Indoors, the inner circle can be outlined with tape or painted with water-based paints on appropriate floor surfaces (so it can be removed later). Outside, the circle can be drawn with white lime or red chalk dust, just as lines are drawn for football and baseball fields. Visibly tracing the circle is important, in order to set up boundaries and to keep dancers from straying into the centre at inappropriate times during the ceremony.

The centre is best marked with a tree, either living in a pot or a cut sapling. We have also experimented with a cairn of stones, a large stump or log, or even an empty chair decorated like a throne, for the unseen Presences to sit upon. The purpose of the centre-piece is to offer a focus for honoring the Goddess and God. It also acts as a focal point for the dancers wishing to make pledges and prayers.

Whether they are held inside or out, the actual layout of the ceremonial grounds is similar for each of my ceremonies. Space permitting, the ground is laid out in a diamond shape, consisting of the four altar shrines placed at the four cardinal points of the compass. The inner circle is then drawn within the diamond, leaving room for the two rings of the yang and yin lines to move between the altars and the inner circle. The inner circle is quartered with different colored strips, pointing to each of the four shrines. (Each element, and each direction, has its own special colors. I use brown and green for North/ Earth, white and yellow for East/Air, red and orange for South/Fire, and blue and purple for West/Water, but other ceremonial systems assign different colors to the elements.) At the very centre is set a tree or some other large, sturdy monument to the Gods. See the diagram in Figure 2.

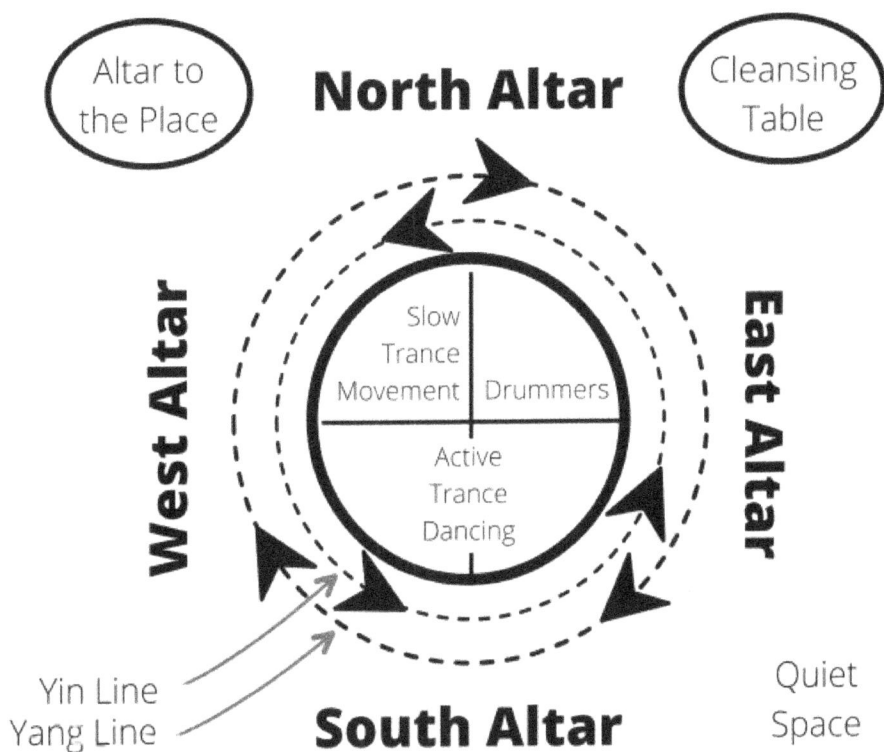

Figure 2: Outdoor or Large Hall Layout

In rectangular halls, or sites that don't have enough room to lay out the altars as I've described above, I modify the design to make the best use of the space available. I may, for instance, put the four shrines in the corners of the room, and draw the inner "circle" as an oval instead. See Figure 3 for this alternative arrangement.

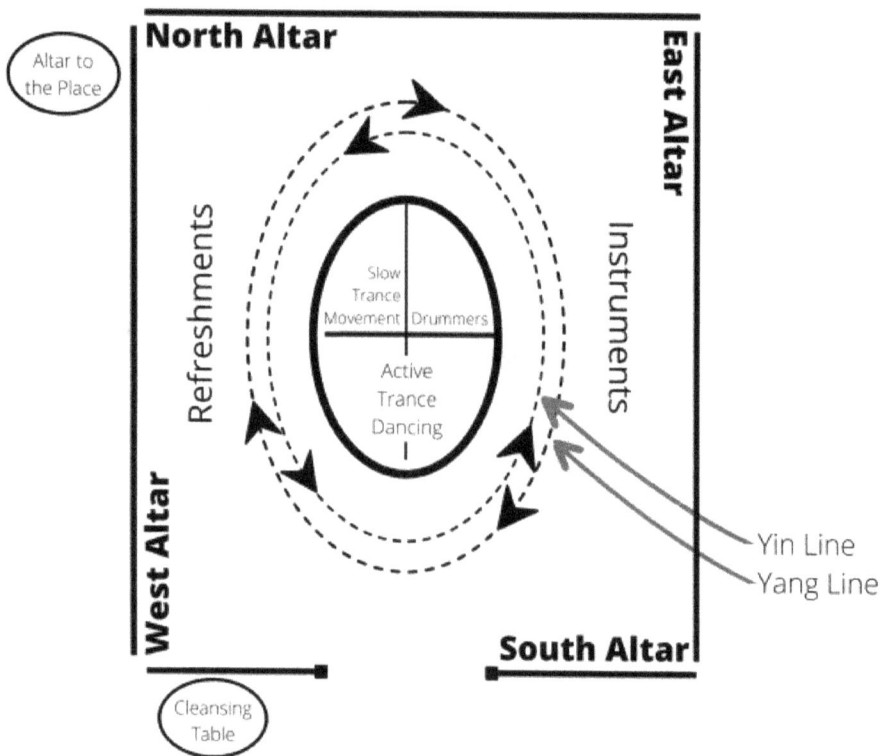

Figure 3: Rectangular Hall Layout

If you are working within a specific ethnic modality you may want to decorate the inner circle with runes or other meaningful symbols. My teacher Elizabeth drew the kabbalist's Tree of Life on the floor of the inner circle. In later versions of the Long Dance when I was reconnecting with my Irish roots I used a S-shaped spiral drawn onto the ground or floor.

For a Samhain rite, when the inner circle is open to dancers, one curve of the spiraling S is a walking meditation symbolizing the participant's descent into the past to seek wisdom from the ancestors. The other curve of the S symbolizes the participant's ascent into the future of the Earth and our descendants, not necessarily biological. We look at our legacy and the wisdom we gain from preparing our world for them.

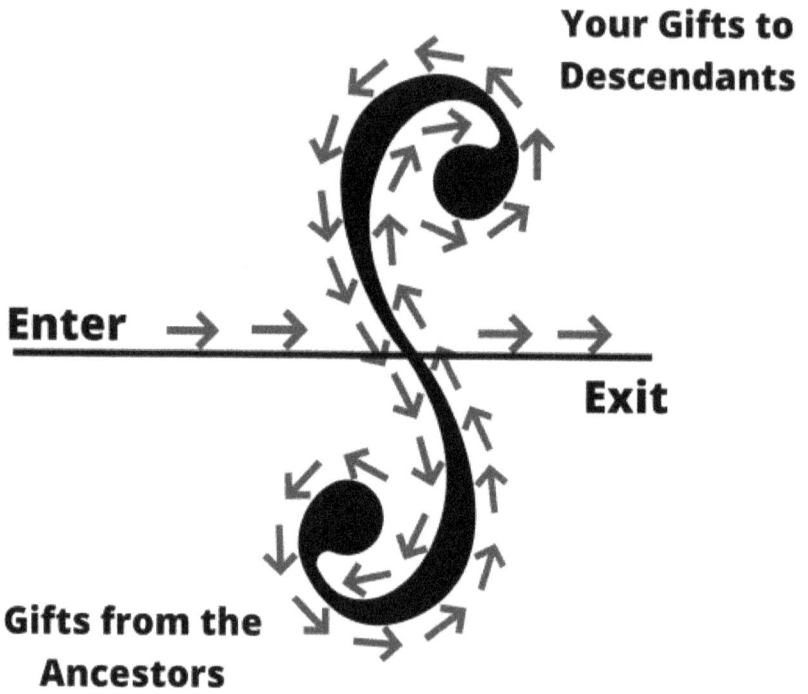

Figure 4: The Celtic spiral layout

Around the edges of the sacred space are other tables set up to hold drums and other instruments, refreshments, and other necessities. Farther out is the Shrine to the Place. In the city, it may not be practical to erect such a shrine, but whenever possible it is a good idea to do so, and to encourage dancers to take quiet time in meditation there whenever they wish.

If a give-away ritual is planned, a table for the give-away items should be put in a conspicuous but safe place. People are expected to lay their gifts upon it (not wrapped), and leave them there until needed. No one is to handle them once they are on the table. During the give-away ceremony itself, the gifts will be brought to the inner circle for the rite. This will be discussed in more detail in a later chapter.

⁊⧉⧈

CEREMONIAL FOODS

Along with creating sacred space, it is necessary to take care of physical needs, and that includes food. I like to keep things simple, so that means a lot of finger foods and simple things like soups and sandwiches made on site. For the feasts, do as much ahead of time as possible, so that everyone can enjoy the ritual without a lot of work. I ask people to bring potluck dishes and nutritious snacks to share that will help cut down on expenses. I also suggest limiting people's intake of coffee. A ritual is not the time to quit an addiction and go through withdrawal symptoms, but juices and herbal teas are a better bet in the long run.

Since managing time is so unpredictable, I prefer to set out a lot of fix-it-yourself foods for most of the meals and snack times. This allows people to follow their own bodily rhythms for eating, and means less fuss for all. Also, everyone should be responsible for cleaning their own place setting; this will help too. Sometimes we have asked people to bring their own breakfast foods, while we provide the rest of the meals. All these are but suggestions that I have found worked, and so I pass them on as that.

For most traditional peoples around the world, the preparing and serving of food at a feast is seen as a sacred duty, not to be treated lightly. With these ancient teachings in mind, participants attending the ceremonials I help organize are asked to see the food they bring in the spirit of a give-away gift.

Food offerings are a way of expressing thankfulness to the Sacred, and of giving service to the community of dancers who take part in the ritual together.

When I began teaching ceremonial, I prepared all the meals myself. I did this because I knew that most of the urban people attending had little awareness of the sacredness of this type of service. There is still a lot of confusion about this act. Many times, participants have offered to cook certain special dishes if the organizers provided the money for the food and other supplies. Once again, here is an example of the confusion that arises as our rituals make the transition from workshop to true religious rite.

In workshops what happens is this: The workshop leader or leaders do all the work of preparation and teaching. In exchange, the attendees compensate them with money. The participants do none of the work, except for following any instructions the leaders give during the workshop. If a participant spends a considerable amount of time preparing food, this is a contribution above and beyond what would normally be expected of him, and naturally he expects to be compensated for it, at least to the extent of having his expenses covered.

This money layout is fine for workshops where the participant plays a more passive role, but in true religious community, this behavior cannot be permitted, because we are all very active parts of the whole. The money collected as an admission charge to a ritual is spent on expenses for the ceremony as a whole, not to pay the leaders (except possibly for a small honorarium).

Money collected should be spent on food prepared by the North Clan (who will often make individual give-away dishes as well), but this North Clan food is intended to be in addition to the contributions of participants, which may not be sufficient for a several-day event. Food is a very sacred offering, and should be seen in that way, and all should share in its preparation as well as its consumption.

We also teach that, when you prepare food for anyone, you treat that task like a meditation, putting good, nourishing thoughts into the food that will be shared in sacred space. (For this reason, I cringe when I hear women advised to take out their anger on their bread dough. What are their families eating?)

At the ceremony, the North Clan takes our extra food offerings and arranges to serve a portion of them at each meal. Before each meal, a prayer is offered to those divine powers that are present at the ceremony. After the grace, a spirit plate is prepared. This plate contains small portions of everything on the table. The plate is then taken outside and given to the spirits, and to any small creatures on the land who might wish to partake of it. After this plate is taken out, the elders are served by younger people at the ceremony, and then the other participants come forward by clan to eat in turn. The purpose here is not one of privilege for any human person, but a way of honoring the ancient wisdom that happens to be within those elders at that time. This, to me, is one of the ways of reclaiming some of our ancient ways.

When I was taught the Long Dance tradition, we served lots of snacks, especially during the all-night dance. At first, I continued that practice, but have now stopped. Serving snacks and teas and coffee during the night only encourages a party atmosphere and acts as a distraction to the true trance process. If there is an ample supper, there is no real need for more nourishment until morning. (For those who have special health requirements, however, such as diabetics, they are expected to do what they need for themselves.) Without being a martyr about it, light fasting can be seen as a part of a dancer's personal pledge during the dance—another way of being challenged.

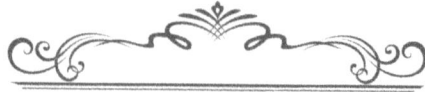

Chapter 4

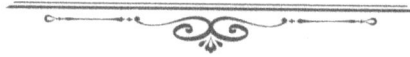

Step 4:
The Cleansing and the Blessing

Cleansing

Cleansing is the most common word used nowadays for this process, but it is perhaps a bit misleading, because, in the sense I am using it, there is no connection with dirt or being unclean. The purpose of this step is really to shift energy patterns. It can be used to move away or break up unwanted vibrations or remnants of past events in places or objects. In human beings, a cleansing is used to shift these energies and make the person more open and accessible to the power and guidance of the Sacred Ones.

In every religion around the world that I can think of, there is always some type of cleansing done. The methods may vary, but the most common types of cleansing used by modern Pagans tend to fall into two groups. The first is the smudge, in which some type of herb or tree resin is burned to create a sweet-smelling smoke. My teachers have claimed that the smoke, when brushed across a person or object, will purify the energy field of unwanted influences that may be hanging on to the person's or object's aura. The smoke is also said to open a person's awareness to the divine powers that are there, waiting for us to tap into them.

Some elders also claim that spirits and ancestors can smell the scents of various herbal smudges, and that they respond differently to different odors. For example, if I was performing a certain ritual evoking Native spirits, I would be wise to use sage or sweetgrass as a smudge, rather than myrrh or frankincense, for these are not herbs that the Native spirits are familiar with.

On the other hand, if I were calling on a Christian saint or a Middle Eastern deity, frankincense would be an excellent herb to use, since both the saint or deity themselves, and the practitioners worshipping them, have used frankincense for many centuries, and the familiar odor would readily act as a trigger to bring about a connection between the deity and the worshippers.

As a rule of thumb, if you wish to use herbs native to your area (which is particularly appropriate if you are invoking the spirits of that area), a good way to find local cleansing smudges is to find herbs that have cleansing properties when used medicinally, as in a tea. These herbs have similar purifying powers when burned as a smudge. Some examples of such plants are sage, cedar, rosemary, pine, artemisia (mugwort), basil, and juniper.

Bear in mind, however, that with smudging, as with other ritual usages, it is not the physical form of the plant itself that is of sole importance. The spiritual essence of a particular plant will add to the work, but it is the power and intent of the person using the smudge that is most important. Both priests and black sorcerers may use the same herbs or other ritual tools; it is their intent and how they use the tools that is significant.

Brushing a person or space is also effective. In the area of the country in which I live cedar boughs are often cut and brushed over a person's body to clear away negative energies. The person doing the brushing often sings as the work is being done. Sometimes a smaller bough is dipped in water and sprinkled for the same effect. I personally find the touch of these sacred boughs very soothing.

Another type of ritual cleansing commonly used is a salt-and-water bath. This may mean an actual bath in water that is dosed with table salt, sea salt or Epsom salts, or it may be only a symbolic sprinkling of the two elements over persons or objects. Teas made from the same cleansing herbs used for smudges (sage, cedar, rosemary, etc.) can also be used for sprinkling or bathing. In addition, tools can be purified by sprinkling them or immersing them in a suitable herbal tea. As with the smudge, the intent is the same, to cleanse away any unwanted presences from the aura and to open the one cleansed to the Sacred.

A variation on this that utilizes the power of water is to immerse oneself in the ocean or a mountain lake or river at either dawn or dusk, depending on the tradition. In the indigenous communities I am aware of, the participants often go in small groups to a secluded place to sing and pray and be renewed. This type of cleansing/blessing can be done before a ceremony or anytime a person feels overwhelmed by modern living and personal or family troubles.

A smudge is a blessing with air and fire; a brushing sprinkling or bathing is a blessing with earth and water. Many people use both methods in a single ritual, to cleanse themselves with all the elements. You could also use one for a cleansing and the other for a blessing; the distinction between cleansing and blessing is described further on in this chapter.

You can use all of these methods interchangeably, depending upon the situation. The point here is not to be rigid about a certain form of cleansing, but to recognize that in some form cleansing is an important part of your preparations. By this act, you open the possibility of a spiritual connection with the divine powers that guide your life. Cleansing should say to the psyche, "I let go of the cares and worries of my everyday life. I set them aside for now, so that I can be more receptive to the influence of the divine."

A further comment about cleansing of a site with the above-mentioned techniques that, if its energy feels really icky, you may want to add, as a first step, before the smudge or sprinkling, sweeping around the perimeter of the space with bundles of thorny plants (such as holly, thistle, or wild rose). As you travel in a counter-clockwise direction around the room, you imagine any unwanted energy patterns clinging to the thorns. When the bundles feel heavy, stop right there and remove them to be burned (away from the site). Begin again at the same spot with a new thorn-bundle, and continue sweeping as before. When the circle has been completed, go back around it clockwise with something (like a herbal smoke) to seal and protect the space.

This is a rather extreme method of cleansing, and if the space is bad enough to need this type of treatment it is probably not suitable for a ritual site anyway, but conditions in the real world are not always ideal, so you may have to use that place and take the best measures you can to make it suitable.

FASTING

There are different types of fasting, depending on your cultural and religious beliefs. To some, fasting means abstaining entirely from food or water for a certain number of days, while for other people, it merely means going without solid food, while continuing to drink water and fruit juices.

Some people consider a fast to be a good way of cleansing and preparing themselves for a ceremony. In moderation I would agree, but for a ritual which involves a lot of strenuous activity, I do not encourage any more than a light fast, one day before the event begins. You will need all your strength to participate fully in the rite.

I know there are many who would not agree with me on this point. Many traditions around the world tend to see the body as dirty, offensive and unclean. For people on these spiritual paths, there is a lot of merit gained, for the individual, and, in some cases, his community, when bodily suffering is endured. I tend to argue for moderation in these matters, because my personal beliefs see value in channeling the spiritual through the physical, rather than in trying to destroy the health of the physical in order to gain the spiritual. This is a personal opinion, however, which may or may not be compatible with your beliefs, dear reader.

BLESSING

When you cleanse a place or even a person, you have created a vacuum. To prevent the area from being recontaminated with another unwanted energy pattern, you need to finish a cleansing and seal it off with a blessing of some sort. Go back over the area just cleansed, imagining the powers of the Divine (however you envision it) entering and protecting the object or place.

For people who have been cleansed just before a ceremony is to begin, the blessing can wait and take place during the ritual rather than immediately after the cleansing. If someone feels very vulnerable, a blessing should be done right away, but normally people should be protected and blessed within the sacred space itself, when the circle is cast. The people responsible for setting up the altars, however, should say a little prayer (a form of blessing) after they are cleansed, before starting their work. This little prayer is needed as a closure, because there is no sacred Circle around them yet for their protection.

Cleansings and blessings often use exactly the same herbs or techniques. The difference between them is the intent. Cleansing is meant to remove existing influences that are not wanted for the work at hand, while blessing is meant to call down the protection and favor of the Divine. Some examples of blessings are prayers, smudges, sprinkling with herbal teas or fresh water (not salt water for a blessing), and drinking juice, wine or tea. If you are using similar techniques for both cleansing and blessing, you need to do them twice – e.g., smudge to cleanse, and then smudge again to bless.

Herbs like cedar, sage, sweetgrass, copal, pine, and other incenses are good things to use for smudge blessings, but they are not the only things available. Do some study to discover what used to be used in your area, or research the tradition in which you are working to bring up other ideas.

At the site of the rituals I direct, we cleanse the area before setting up the altars and making a sacred space. The clan leaders, and anyone else handling the items for the altars, need also to cleanse and ground themselves before beginning their work. After all is in order and the altars have been set up, we go back over the area with a smudge and a prayer for the health and protection of all within the energy circle of the ceremony.

⌾∞

GROUNDING AND CENTERING

Though the term "grounding" may not be used outside of Wiccan or New Age groups, every spiritual discipline around the world that I know of uses some method of focusing and centering the energy in the body and the present moment. To do spiritual work, it is necessary not only to cleanse oneself, but to set aside mundane reality and step into the realm of the Sacred where anything is possible. It is very important in doing this to be fully "present" in the moment (both in body and mind). The practitioner must be very aware of the self and the seen and unseen forces around him or her.

Grounding and centering is more than this, however. It is an opening of the self to the spirit realm. It is allowing the self to become a channel through which the unseen forces can work without draining the life force of the person doing the channeling. You have to establish a strong link between yourself and the Earth, which includes being very present in your body, and opening up an energy cord down to the Earth.

How do you ground yourself? The simplest way is to use a technique of deep breathing, combined with an opening of the crown and base chakras, to create an open flow of energy between the spirits of Earth and Sky. To do this, you visualize a cord descending from the base of your spine into the Earth, through which you can draw up fresh vital force and discharge stale energy, and then open the crown of your head to the Sky and draw down additional power from the heavens.

Some people liken this technique to the effect of a lightning rod during a storm. When doing spiritual work of any kind, you need to tap into a lot of energy for it to be effective. This energy is readily available from the Universe around us, as well as being present in our own bodies. However, we want to avoid either draining our own reserves or being consumed by an excess of external force. Therefore, we can open ourselves to incoming energy from Earth and Sky (so as not to use up our own), and then drain the excess down into the Earth whenever needed, especially at the completion of the rite.

Centering is a little different from grounding. When you ground yourself, you draw in energy from outside yourself. When you center, you connect yourself to your own internal sources of power. One way to do it is to bring your awareness to the center of your body, the point the Chinese call the tan tien. This is approximately the center of gravity of your body, a point two to three fingers' width below the navel and then two to three fingers' width toward the backbone. (This locating technique works better on relatively thin people.) For women, the center is in approximately the same place as the womb. Another way of centering is to pay attention to your breath, and to follow it until it becomes deep and slow and unobstructed. You can also combine the two techniques by "breathing into your tan tien."

Spiritual work takes place in a separate reality, which is very ethereal. If you are not connected to the Earth and centered in your body during this work, you may reach the point where you dwell permanently in this separate reality. You will then become progressively more unbalanced, perhaps even to the point of madness. Our challenge in being born into this world is to combine our spirituality with our physical reality, rather than attempting to live entirely in either the mundane or the ethereal realm.

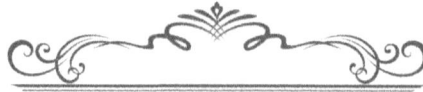

Chapter 5

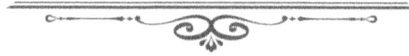

Step 5:
The Opening of the Ritual

Casting the Circle

Circle casting is used by pagans and other indigenous traditions to define the sacred space in which a ritual will take place. The divine forces raised within a ritual are concentrated in one area by the Circle, and without that confinement, the energy would immediately dissipate before the power could build to a point where it could be used for spiritual or healing purposes. The Circle also serves to protect the participants from unwanted or harmful energies that may be attracted to the working. Furthermore, when a Circle is cast, the act of casting it clearly designates the beginning of a ritual, and dispelling the Circle equally clearly designates the end – thus defining the limits of the ritual in time as well as in space.

In traditions like Christianity or Buddhism, this step may not be so emphasized, because there is usually a church or temple that has been especially constructed and dedicated for the purpose of ritual and so becomes a permanent place of worship and an open channel to the Divine. Most Earth-centered religions don't build churches, so the spots chosen by these groups may be used for other functions or may be part of the natural world, and therefore need to be redefined each time a ceremony is held.

Originally, around the world certain springs, rock formations, or groves of trees were used by Indigenous people for worship. A few of them have survived to modern times—and are still in use. Over time, Pagan groups in North America may be able to rediscover or establish more of such places. However, it's a good idea, even in a known sacred space, to cast a Circle for protection as well as to define each ritual in time and space.

For the purpose of a modern Pagan ceremonial, a Circle is usually cast by surrounding the ritual space with a ring of protection (often the imagery of white light or fire), and then inviting the elemental guardians of the four directions and the presiding Gods to participate in, witness, and keep safe the rites about to begin. In the ceremonies that I perform, the elders or the keepers of the four sacred shrines invite the guardians of the directions to enter, either by chanting and drumming, by a special dance, or by a prayer to honor and acknowledge their presence. The Gods or Goddesses invoked in the Centre of the Circle are invited and honored in a similar manner.

The point to keep in mind here is that the Circle is not a flat circle, but more like a sphere or the shell of an egg, enclosing the sacred space above and below the participants as well. Many beginners don't know that the Circle is actually a sphere or forget to visualize it that way, and thus leave a portion of their workings unprotected.

Sometimes the Circle is cast by one or more of the leaders, with a door left open to admit the rest of the participants afterward, but the more common way is to bring everyone into the space and then cast the Circle around them. In Pagan terms, entering a Circle (or casting it around you) is called "stepping between the worlds," which is a way of acknowledging an altered state of consciousness in which anything can happen without challenging one's sanity.

Since a Circle is an energy field that defines and protects a space, it is important to be conscious of breaking that field if you need to leave the Circle once it is cast. You can visualize yourself opening a gate in the Circle and then closing it behind you, so the protective sphere remains intact. With some workings or especially serious parts of long rituals, you need to be very strict about not leaving the Circle and thus breaking the energy flow (even with a gate), but for others we try to imagine the Circle cast around the entire site to make it easy to move about and still remain within the protected space.

Many people, because of their lack of experience, don't take the Circle very seriously, but when it is cast properly, by a powerful individual or group, you should actually feel a tingling if you cross the Circle without making a gate. Also, crossing the Circle in this way is likely to reduce the effectiveness of the work, since a damaged Circle is less efficient at containing and concentrating power.

INVOKING THE DEITIES

Now the opening is done, and who of the Sacred Ones are asked to attend will set the tone and colour for the entire event. I believe it is important to define, not only the Circle, but the type of energies with which you wish to work. For that reason, it is important to take some care in your planning of this step, in deciding which deity or deities to summon.

In a ceremony lasting several days, it is possible to use several types of castings and invocations, some more elaborate than others. Each day may begin with a re-establishment of the Circle and a re-invocation of the Deities. Also, different Gods might be summoned on different days, to guide separate phases of the ritual. I do suggest that the first invocation, or the major one, be very dramatic, with the power to evoke a lot of feeling-energy in the participants' response. This means allowing some of your more experienced members to perform this act, for it is the strength and power of the human will that can pull in the spiritual forces needed to perform successful ritual. Here once again, I will stress the importance of focus, and not allowing idle chatter or distracting movement to disrupt the energy flow and concentration of the participants.

Whatever archetypal energies, Gods, or Goddesses you wish to invoke to witness and bless your rites should be called in after defining your sacred space. The deities from above and below are called to the Centre of the Circle, thus forming a globe or sphere rather than a flat surface in which to work.

Which tradition you are working in will determine how many deities you chose to invite into your sacred space, whether one, or two, or many. Some Pagan traditions invoke the Goddess of the Earth and the God of the Heavens to represent the directions of above and below, but this is totally arbitrary, and can be done in other ways. Other Pagans regard all deities as aspects of the One Divine, and may invite only that One, or may summon as many aspects of the One as seem appropriate for the work. Also, some people choose to invite a deity for each direction, whereas I tend to see the spirits of the directions as elemental forces rather than specific Gods or Goddesses.

THE STATEMENT OF INTENT

This statement says to all who have come together (physical and spiritual, seen and unseen) what you intend to do in this rite and how you intend to do it. ("We are gathered here together to unite this man and this woman in holy matrimony" is a good example of one type of statement of intent.) Statements of intent are often left out of New Age rituals because the people performing them don't always have a clear idea of what they are doing and why they are doing it. The statement of intent is a way to focus on why you are there at the ritual and what you hope to accomplish. It lets everybody, both divine archetype and human, know what's going on and what to expect.

At my rituals, we make the statement of intent in a couple of ways. The wise elder outlines to the witnesses and the participants what will be going on during the time we are together. Also, at the opening council (which is described later in this chapter), participants will be given time to say what they personally want to give and receive from the ritual; this is another way of stating intent.

A personal pledge made at this time has far more meaning than something spoken at other times, because it is sworn in ritual space with the unseen Powers of the Sacred as witnesses. Any statement made within the Sacred Circle has far-reaching echoes for your well-being, so have a care what is spoken or sworn to during such a time. (See the discussion of personal pledges in Chapter 2 – The Preparation of a Ceremony.)

A physical symbol can be used to represent a pledge, often long after the words have been spoken and the ceremony ended. If you keep the physical object and put it where you will see it, then every time it catches your eye it will remind you to focus on your commitment, or on the work that is still being done by the ritual that you performed. When your promises have been fulfilled and the work is completed, then dispose of the physical object in some appropriate manner.

In my rituals, along with vocalizing a statement of intent or a pledge, we often hang ribbons on the centre pole, to represent in a very physical way what has been said. In this way, it is not forgotten; each time a dancer looks to the centre pole, he or she sees the ribbon as a reminder of their words. This adds power to the intention, by increasing the energy focused upon it. After the event, these ribbons can be disposed of in several ways: burned, buried, put in the ocean, or left in a safe spot to blow in the wind. Whatever is done, it is important to make some type of ending (i.e., to dispose of the ribbons in some way), to complete what you have begun.

$$\otimes$$

THE OPENING COUNCIL

As I perform it in my rituals, this Council is a very structured affair, in which a symbol such as a stick, a feather, a crystal, or a bowl of water is passed around the circle. While the object is being passed, only the person holding it has the right to speak. Participants are asked a short list of specific questions, such as "Who are you? What do you do in the world? What do you hope to get from this experience, and what are you willing to give in return?" As the talking-stick (or other symbol) is passed, the questions are repeated by each member so that we stay on track. That is, the person who has just answered the questions asks them again of the next speaker.

With between twenty and fifty people to speak, a time limit of three minutes per person is imposed. Someone keeps time with a stop watch and rings a little bell when the time for each speaker is up. It is important to make sure that people are actually sitting in a circle or an oval, so that everyone can see everyone else and hear clearly what is being said.

The primary purpose of the Opening Council is to give each participant a chance to speak to the group as a whole. It helps the group to bond and to get to know one another. Members may use this time to state, or re-state, their personal pledges. The Council is also a good time for the elders to give general teachings and establish the focus of the event.

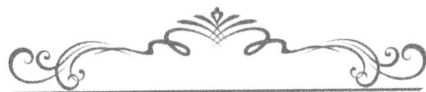

Chapter 6

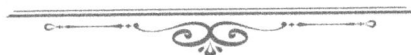

Step 6:
The Body of the Ritual

What I am referring to by the term "body" is that main portion of a ritual in which the actual work of the ceremony is done. This is the process of raising energy and directing it to fulfil the purpose of the rite. In most books I have read on the subject of ritual, there is a great amount of detail spent on directions for the opening step of a rite, but after that things tend to get a bit vague. This is understandable, because each ritual will have its own purpose, and thus need different activities to achieve its goals. What I can offer here are some suggestions on methods of raising and channeling energy that may add depth and resonance to your ceremonial workings. Some of this material comes from my Native background, and some from my experience with the Long Dance ceremonial and other European traditions. The information that follows may offer you a different perspective in which to design your own ceremonial style.

THE HUMAN VOICE

For many modern people, using the human voice effectively is a lost art. Rare is the person who does not use radio, TV, Spotify, or some other kind of digital recording device to make his music. We rely on mechanical aids to create entertainment that would have been done by real people in former times. Most of us have forgotten what a wonderful tool the human voice really is. I mean the voice of ordinary people, not just people who have an extraordinary natural singing talent. With only minimal training and practice, plus the confidence to use it fully, your own voice can become one of your most important magical tools. The ability of the voice to express emotions is of the utmost importance when doing any type of ceremonial or magical work.

Most New Age circles, especially women's circles, have little understanding of how to use the voice effectively. What comes out of the mouth when asked to chant or sing is this faint, squeaky little sound that can barely be heard in the next room. Unfortunately, the whole point is to be heard, both by the other participants and by the Divine. How well you are able to project power through your vocal cords usually says a lot about how grounded and comfortable you are with yourself and the deities you honor. (This does not apply, of course, if you have a physical disability that prevents you from using your voice in a normal manner.)

The reasons for this lack of self-confidence in using the voice are various, but it is an issue we need to look at when studying the ritual arts. For many women, and some men, loud, forceful voices are equated with abuse and aggression. To avoid becoming victims, they have trained themselves since childhood to speak as quietly as possible, so as not to be noticed or hurt.

Others don't wish to speak out because all their lives they have been criticized and put down, so that now they are afraid of failure or appearing foolish in front of others, and thus inviting more criticism and self-blame. This is a terrible tragedy, for the voice is a great channel of power in a ritual, as well in our daily lives.

Part of the planning and group sessions held leading up to a ceremonial event should be creating and practicing songs and chants that belong to that ceremony itself, kept to sing only at that ceremony or other sacred events. These can be prayer songs developed and sung by the whole or part of the group, or songs created by an individual as a personal song to be sung at the event, by the person, or by others while the person dances.

For those of us who physically can't speak, or can't speak clearly, there are alternatives. Movement and dance, as well as other art forms, can channel the energies of the Universe equally well. But it will be up to the physically-challenged individual to adapt to his or her own limitations in whatever ways are necessary. For the rest of us who only have mental or emotional blocks to overcome, a combination of therapy, voice training, and practice can break down these blocks, or at least minimize their effects.

As any actor or voice teacher will tell you, the secret behind the effective use of the voice is the breath. Most people breathe very shallowly, from the chest cavity alone. This type of breathing puts a lot of strain on the vocal cords when singing or speaking. It can never produce the full, rich tones that can be achieved with a deep breath coming all the way from the belly and releaced slowly as sound. When you ground and centre yourself, and breathe the air down into your belly and then relcase it, you are drawing in the sacred life-force and mixing it with the essence of your own being. This is a powerful magical gift. To speak or sing is, in magical terms, to create, and to speak or sing with power and passion is to add much more to that creation.

It can be a question of attitude as well as training. If you don't allow your ego to get involved, but see yourself rather as a channel to be used by the deities you honor, you can divorce yourself from a lot of embarrassment and insecurity that would be present if the ego ran the show. Don't waste the energy worrying about how you appear to others, but instead concentrate on your connection with the unseen forces of the Sacred that you have a desire to communicate with. I also suggest that the serious student of ritual get some acting training. There are many practical skills to be learned from the theatre, for its ancient roots began in religious ritual. (We will discuss the theatre in more detail later on.)

In other cultures around the world, people understand the power inherent in the voice. In most martial arts, the voice is uscd to direct the power of the punch or throw. There are stories of old masters being able to kill small animals through the power of their voices alone. In parts of Africa, the Middle East and North America, women made (and still make) an ululating cry with such force that they can use it for their own protection, or to encourage their men going into battle. Through toning and song, the voice also has the power to heal and foster health and well-being. All these examples point to the importance of the human voice throughout our history, and why we cannot ignore its training and power in our modern technological age.

CHANTING AND SONG

To me, a song is a melody with words that are laid out in verses. These verses may tell a story or have a repetitious chorus, but they are seldom very long in duration. Chants, on the other hand, are a short melody with short phrases or wordless vocalizations that can be repeated over and over endlessly to produce a light trance state. All over the world, songs and chants are used as a vital part of most ceremony and ritual. Music in general, and the voice in particular, has the power to stimulate certain emotional or healing states within the human body. This can be a powerful force when directed through the medium of a ritual. There is power in the human voice even for the listener, but different, and perhaps much greater, power for those actually singing.

In the Long Dance ceremony, we use songs or chants at the beginning and ending of the event. These chants, with simple, easily-learned words, can bring people together and help them focus on the business at hand. Songs set the mood and tone, and if they are only half-heartedly sung they can affect the quality of the work to be done, so it is important to start off well.

During the body of the ceremony, especially during the trance dance itself, we use only chants that are vocalized sounds, not sung with words at all. There is an important reason for this. When you are deepening into the trance state, your brain needs to go back to an older, more reptilian way of responding to stimuli. In this instance, vocalizations can add feeling to the movements of the dance, without engaging the conscious mind in the active processing of the meanings of words. When words are sung, the mind snaps back to conscious awareness, as it tries to make sense of what it is hearing. This can be like a slap of cold water in the face when a dancer is just sinking into trance.

The person is rudely jerked back to a conscious state of awareness. For this reason, I suggest the use of vocalizations rather than chants or songs with words. Similarly, I suggest that the tune of the vocalizations not be similar to that of any known song that has words. If the melody reminds the dancers of some existing song, their minds will try to put the remembered (or poorly-remembered) words to the tune. This will jerk them back to conscious awareness as shockingly as hearing actual words. This is why I stress creating chants and songs for certain rites specifically to avoid other associations.

In keeping with this topic there is a variation of the vocalized chant used by some indigenous peoples and others called,"the call and response." The stomp dance music of the Iroquois and the tribes of the south east like the Creek and

Cherokee are good examples of this type of music. In call and response, there is a lead singer who chants a phrase which is then repeated by the other drummers or even all the participants, depending on the context. Pow wow drum songs are similar as well. The lead usually changes from song to song or even within the song itself sometimes.

Many people don't realize that much of Native American dance music is vocalized sounds, rather than songs sung in a particular language. The music creates and expresses a feeling without being confined by the limitations of words.

For this same reason, I end a ritual with songs or chants that do contain words. The words will help bring people out of trance and back to the reality of the moment. When ending a rite, it is important to ground yourself (draining off excess energy into the Earth) and be very clear about where you are, and that you are functioning normally and are capable of coping with traffic and other problems in the outside world. Song can help dancers to focus and can re-structure group unity as well, which is why I use it to begin and end a rite.

One of the strongest pulls, for me personally, to go back to Native ceremonials is the music. Nothing I have heard in Western European music has the power to move me like Native music can. This is a personal bias, but I also feel that it is time we reclaim the vital force to be found in our ancient healing music, whatever part of the world we come from.

Adding to this thought, I have found some pagan music from Europe recently that comes pretty close to what I'm talking about. This is the songs labled Northern Spirit on some of the music streaming services. Though the chants are modified for their entertainment value, and I can't speak a word of the languages they are sung in, I can still tell by the song's structure if it is a pagan religious chant, a bard's ballad, or something else. Some other examples of powerful ways to use the human voice are various types of throat singing practiced by the Inuit, Tibetan and Mongolian singers. Their techniques take a lot of practice and often years to perfect, so they aren't included in this book, but they are well worth the effort if you can find a teacher.

We need to find guidelines in older cultures to recreate our own healing and ritual music for today. To do this, we must first understand that music has a different function in other parts of the world than it does in modern societies. Most of modern music is designed for entertainment alone. For this reason, harmony takes precedence over melody. (By harmony, I mean voices and instruments playing several harmonious notes at once, rather than all singing a single note at a time. Even *acapella* music usually has several singers harmonizing instead of singing in unison.)

With this type of music, the arrangement and back-up is very important, and needs constant variation throughout the piece to hold the listeners' and performers' interest. Words are used to make a statement, and the inflection of an individual singer's voice is what conveys emotion. Two modern singers can sing the same song and create very different feelings, whereas in traditional music sung in the old ways, two singers singing the same thing will convey the same feeling, since it is inherent in the tones of the music itself.

Sometimes traditional music is meant to be monotonous, and often it is sung using a different scale that may seem out of tune to the Western, European-trained, ear. One of the great personal tragedies for me is how Native and, to a lesser extent, old Celtic and Norse music is changing due to the influence of modern music. Old Native music is sung in a different tonal scale than the European do re mi scale. When I hear West Coast and Celtic elders sing, I hear the sounds of wind and rain blowing through the trees. When the Dene of the Northwest Territories sing, I feel the pulse of the hooves of caribou running across frozen tundra. Each culture's music is very different, and it takes time, skill, and immersion in a culture to reproduce the songs right.

When I have heard non-Natives singing what they thought was Native music, it never sounded right, because unconsciously they would change the tunes to fit the modern do re mi scale. The original melody would seem off-key to them after years of being bombarded by pop tunes on radio and TV.

I used to think that white people didn't have a good ear, and were copying the sounds poorly. Now I know that is not necessarily so. They sing the way their Native teachers (who are mostly young or middle-aged) have taught them. Those Natives who have grown up with a lot of urban influence don't hear the old songs correctly either. I try to comfort myself with the reminder that change is a part of all life, but I still indulge in a tear of sadness at times for what is being lost.

In most other parts of the world, more emphasis is placed on the melody and on a simple, rhythmic or repetitive background sound or drone (such as bagpipes, mismars, drums, or gongs). Harmony and fancy arrangements are only used when there is an attempt to make this music more palatable to modern taste.

The trick, for us, is to re-create the essence of the music, not to parrot other cultures' forms. What function does music play in a ritual or in the society in general? That is what needs to be re-created, not actual songs taken out of their cultural context.

An example of what not to do is how Native American music is commonly treated by the New Age. As I mentioned earlier, Native music is usually sung on a pentatonic scale, which means it sounds flat or off-key to the uninstructed ear. Modern singers usually make an attempt to memorize the words or vocalizations and to reproduce them correctly, but the melody of the chant usually ends up sounding like an opera aria or a romantic love song, since those are the closest models of singing most of us are familiar with. It is not only whites, but urbanized Natives, who sing this music incorrectly, because, being away from their Native cultural roots, they lack the traditional training and the sensitivity of ear to sing it properly.

Native music is also meant to be monotonous, with little or no emphasis or inflection. Most modern singers are so used to rock music that they get bored and try to jazz up the songs, which in turn changes their purpose from healing, trance-invoking music to music fit only for entertainment. In the context of entertainment, we are used to praising singers for putting their personal stamp on an old song, but ritual music ought not to have the mark of individuality on it. That is for stroking the singer's ego, not for aiding dancers to go into trance or pleasing the Goddesses and Gods.

We are used to hearing songs lasting perhaps 5 minutes, at most. When we hear a longer piece, we very quickly get bored and start looking for variety. Yet monotony is the very purpose of most ritual music, since when the conscious mind is sufficiently bored, it eventually turns itself off and goes away for a while, leaving the person in a timeless, wordless state of consciousness or light trance, which allows spiritual revelation and healing to take place.

There is a special timbre and quality to the voice that, it could be argued, is intrinsic to different cultural and racial groups. This quality, combined with the use of different melodic scales, gives music its cultural and racial resonance. These sounds, in turn, have the ability to stimulate certain racial memories. When used correctly by indigenous singers, where the quality of the voice matches the tone of the music, it can be a powerful experience for others of the same culture.

This is not an easy concept to explain, and many would disagree with me. I can only say that, from my own experience, it seems to be true. When I listen to a certain type of old Celtic or Norse chant, sung by a knowledgeable elder, I feel something that I feel from no other music. The same is true for me when I hear old people sing some Native songs.

The point I am trying to make here is to advise you not to go out and blindly copy another's culture and songs because that tradition is more easily accessible than your own ancient roots, but to take the time and study to find out what resonates for you, and work on from there. In the long run, this will have much more meaning for you.

I understand that most people's resistance to this idea is very strong and comes from low self-esteem and cultural guilt. These are very real problems, but they must be looked at honestly and worked with, in order to have some balance and well-being in one's personal religious practice.

⊙≫≪

SACRED VERSUS FOLK Music

The difference between sacred and folk music is little understood by modern peoples. Folk music, as its name implies, is music that belongs to the people (the folk). It can be sung by anyone, anywhere and at any time. Sacred music, on the other hand, is always "owned," by a person, a group, or a ceremony. The force and power of sacred music is determined by how it is used and on what occasions it is sung.

Sacred music should never be taken out of context, for fear it will lose its vital force. An example of this kind of devaluing is the Christmas carol. For hundreds of years, these beautiful songs were sung only around Christmas-time. No one would dream of singing them in July—or even October, for example; it just wouldn't seem right. This is a good example of sacred music that is owned by a seasonal ceremony, rather than by a particular person or persons.

So, because these songs were linked to a certain ceremonial event, they had a lot of power to move the hearts of the people who share the Christian faith and who sing or hear them. The old carols were sung simply, and had the power to inspire generosity, love, and a desire for peace on Earth. (By the "old carols," I mean the old sacred songs, like *Silent Night*, *The First Noel*, or *We Three Kings*, rather than modern schlock like *Frosty the Snowman*.) Unfortunately for the carols, they have been taken over and commercialized (in stores and on radio and TV) to the point that they, like so much of modern life, are becoming sterile and meaningless.

In traditional Native society, ritual music is never taken lightly. All sacred music belongs to someone, and cannot be used by another person, or in another context, without the permission of its owner. Using another person's music can be an even most serious offense than stealing is in our society, since the music is psychically linked to the person who owns it, and evil sorcerers who learn the music can use it to curse the rightful owner.

Like the carol in earlier times (which was owned by the Christmas season), the ownership principle is what has enabled indigenous sacred music to maintain its vitality throughout the centuries. The music is seen as having a power and a living spirit of its own, and so is treated with respect.

I cringe when I attend a New Age rite and someone pipes up with something like "I learned this song at the sweat-lodge last week, and I'll sing it for you right now." I am not trying to run down these well-meaning people's motivations. They have had a beautiful experience, and may sincerely want to share something of the power of that event with others. The problem is that they are taking a song out of context, and also that they may not have the permission of the owner to sing that song.

In addition, they are robbing both the music and its audience of the chance at some later time to experience the song in its proper setting. Whatever the reason, the point is still that to use sacred music in this way drains its power and brings it down to the realm of the folk song.

Some of the most beautiful and moving New Age sacred music has gone down this road. These pieces are sung anywhere, anytime, and sometimes I think I'm going to scream if I hear them one more time, because they have been so misused and abused.

I know many workshop facilitators who have agreed to share and tape their chants. There is a lot of pressure to do this, from students who are starving for something sacred. Perhaps some chants have been channeled just for the purpose of being used in a folk-song way, to help raise awareness. I have shared a couple of chants for this purpose myself after long consideration, but I also believe that part of our spiritual training must be to create for ourselves a type of sacred music that reflects our individual and group experience as well as the land where we live.

Our modern society has grown lazy; radio and CDs have robbed us of our creativity, and it's time to renew those old connections. (I would also be happy to hear different songs in different parts of the country, instead of mass media uniformity.)

I also take issue with recording these songs in fancy high-tech arrangements that are great for sitting around your living room entertaining your friends with, but that are afterwards relatively sterile, in the spiritual sense, when brought back to the Sacred Circle, because they have acquired secular connotations from being heard outside of a ritual context. Some groups even use taped chants in their rituals, believing that the music recorded in professional studios is "better" than anything they can do themselves. It may indeed be better, in a technical, though not a magical, sense; it may even be "perfect." All you have to put up against the sterile electronic perfection of recorded music is your passion and your humanity, but that beats perfection hands down anytime.

Many would argue that New Age people need to know these songs in order to re-establish the Old Religion, and that the best way to do that is to make the music available to everyone. Once I agreed with that argument, but I now believe this is a mistake. Mass production and distribution is not the answer. Sacred music needs to come from within, and it needs to belong to someone human, deity, or ceremony if it is to grow and remain strong.

It is OK to have special or even secret sacred music that belongs only to those who create and sing it. Tapping into our racial and cultural roots, this music is our link with the past and our legacy to the future, so let's treat it with honor and respect.

Through centering and meditation, the Gods themselves will direct you in the creation of sacred music. With patience and time, you will have all that you need. You may also receive guidance from spirits dwelling within special instruments. I have had the experience of possessing certain instruments that have come to me in a sacred way, and that have taught me their sacred songs.

I learned them by centering myself and opening myself up to the music within these instruments.

⚬〰〰

THE SACRED DRUM

The old people say that the drum is the heartbeat of the people. Of all the musical instruments invented by humankind, the drum is one of the oldest and most sacred. There is a power in the drum that even today attracts people like a magnet, whenever it is played.

It is important to honor the sacredness of the drum, and to teach a certain amount of drum etiquette at these seasonal rituals. I teach that the East Clan leader is in sole charge of the drum during the ceremonial event. This means that no one picks up a drumstick or goes near the main drum or drums without that person's permission. This may sound like a bit of power tripping to the uninformed, but let me assure you that it is not. The East Clan elder has a great spiritual responsibility that cannot be taken lightly. Much of the power generated during the rite depends on the drum.

In some cases this may mean that only the East Clan members drum for the night; in other cases, if the East Clan is weak in experienced people, it may mean that other clan members help out, under the guidance of the East Clan leader. I can't stress enough that, like all the clan leadership, the people who take on these duties have chosen this as their act of service to the Sacred and to the community. This usually means that they give up the luxury of just relaxing and flowing with the process of the ceremony. Such service has its rewards, but it is a very different experience, and so deserves respect from the other participants.

Getting back to the drum and its etiquette, it is important to allow the East Clan to do their job. Never is a dancer permitted to tell that clan leader what to do. Through spiritual guidance, the East elder will be given directions on what is needed.

One of the ways that some groups have chosen to encourage this reverence for the drums and their players is to pay honor to the drums, by filing past them, offering a prayer of thanks, and either bowing to the drums or kissing them, both at the beginning and the ending of the rite. I agree with this practice, and encourage it in my work.

I use the drum as a background sound to almost everything I do in the ceremonial circle. With simple repetitious rhythms, I allow the body to relax and flow with its feelings. In the Long Dance, as I was taught it by Elizabeth Cogburn, we use a 1-1-1-1 rhythm with no accents on any of the beats. This is the basic heartbeat of the dance. Its simple, repetitive pulse tends to lead participants into a light trance. Groups I work with have also experimented with congas and other hand drums during rituals, but these drums and their alternative rhythms must always be subordinate to, and in sync with, the dominant 1-1-1-1 beat.

The purpose of the drum is to involve the body, and thus the whole being, in the transformation process. Different rhythms, like different sounds, affect the body in different ways. The basic 1-1-1-1 beat is a simple one that, over time, allows the mind to wander far away from the simple movements that the body may be doing to this beat. This can be used as a form of meditation, to achieve guidance and enlightenment.

The rhythms produced by the conga drums, on the other hand, bring the centre of concentration very strongly back to the body. This can mean that if a person is uncomfortable with their body, especially their sexual body, or if the conga rhythms are alien to their own natural and cultural resonances, they may find the rhythms of the congas very upsetting, while others present at the same dance may revel in the feeling of being totally alive and present in their bodies. The goal of your ceremonial work should determine what type of music you use. Ask yourselves what effect you wish to achieve.

A word of caution: simple rhythms that everyone can follow and play are best for most ceremonial work. For certain portions of the rite (such as the sacred theatre), it would be okay to use a special rhythm that only a few can play, but what is never okay is the carried-away, beatnik type of drumming where the drummer goes berserk on the bongos. This kind of solo performance is fine on stage, but not in a rite where everyone is trying to work together and blend into one. Such grandstanding may be very satisfying to the drummer, but is totally out of sync with the rest of the dancers and musicians. I find this wild drumming is usually a problem only when drugs or alcohol are used by the participants.

I ask that all drummers stay together in one quarter of the inner circle; this prevents the sound field from becoming unclear, because all the drummers are close enough to see and hear one another. I also suggest that no more than four or five drummers play at any one time; this will also help to keep the sound field clean. (By a "clean sound field", I mean that all the drums beat at precisely the same moment.) It can be easier for all the drums to stay together on the beat if the drummers know that one drum is dominant, and keep their eyes on that drummer. A simple trick to focus is for the lead drummer to tie a red ribbon around his/her drumstick, making it easier to follow by the other drummers.

Each group may work out their own system, but a technique that I have used for relieving drummers is, when a particular drummer gets tired, that person holds his or her drumstick in the air, and that's a signal for someone else to take a turn on the drum.

The simple 1-1-1-1 rhythm is easy to learn, so everyone can take a turn at the drums, but the one thing that is hard for beginners to learn is not to accent any of the beats. The simple beat appears too monotonous, so there is a strong tendency to want to jazz it up, to fit the ideas of modern music. In this case, however, the effect that we are striving for is monotony, which will foster the trance state. Dancers may wish to carry rattles and other small hand instruments (such as finger cymbals or soft bells) with them as they move around the circle. These and other instruments are a welcome addition to the drums' throbbing beat.

At our dances, anyone wishing to sing (in vocalized sounds only) stands near the drummers. This will get the attention of other participants, who may wish to join in the chant, either by coming to stand by the lead singer or by chanting as they move about the floor. Another possibility is to use a simple phrase, such as "Hai-ya" or "Hai-yo", that the yang and yin lines chant throughout the dance. In that case, what those sounds are doing is acting as an aid for the dance steps, to help keep the rhythm going. After a time, the sounds become like a mantra, and help the dancers to go into trance.

Don't be rigid about the yang and yin rings' chants, because at some point in the dance, someone may wish to channel a vocalized chant that would be inhibited if the yin and yang sounds are too dominant. These channeled sounds are important, because they may evolve into ceremonial chants that will be used from year to year, and will belong to the seasonal ceremony itself, or they may be individuals' personal songs; in either case, they should be encouraged within the dance.

My last thought concerning the drum, or any other instrument used for ritual, for that matter, is that these things are sacred and need to be treated with respect. If you are careful with your power objects, a spirit will come to dwell in them. This spirit power can offer you guidance and enlightenment if it is taken care of and treated well. I have discussed this at greater length in Chapter 2, but it bears repeating here.

If you want your things to keep their power, then you must be very careful how and who handles them. Never leave them lying around for anyone (including children) to handle or treat disrespectfully. To be the keeper of a sacred drum is to take on a responsibility to the spirit of that drum, and that should be taken seriously, for you are now a channel for the power of a ritual to work through. Often these sacred items will tell you their personal names. These names are a thing of power that should not be given out lightly to others, lest the power of the object be drained by the inappropriate use of its name. These are a few of the teachings I was given by the elders, and so I pass them on to those who may not be fortunate enough to have learned such things yet.

⚬❧

SACRED DANCE

After five to seven minutes of any repetitious activity, the conscious mind gets bored with its task, and its attention begins to wander. Anyone who has tried to master an Oriental meditation technique can testify to the fact that it takes a lot of discipline and concentration to channel the mind into the meditative pathways in which you wish it to travel.

In many schools of religious study, the way to enlightenment is by overcoming and transcending the body and our physical reality. The physical world is seen as an illusion from which we must obtain release in order to achieve true spirituality. This is the fundamental teaching of both Christian and most Eastern religions.

There are, however, other spiritual paths, less well-known, that choose an alternative means of enlightenment. In these traditions, it is seen as a great privilege to be born into the physical world. To be able to experience life through the senses is a wondrous blessing, not to be dismissed or taken lightly. These paths pursue enlightenment and transformation by immersing the self in the physical plane, rather than trying to escape it. (I am not talking about self-indulgence or debauchery here.) One such path is sacred dance, which is a style of movement and dance in which the body is used in such a way as to bring about change and spiritual transformation. With dance, one can "move" through a problem, releasing old traumas stored within the body tissues, thus enabling the whole being to be a part of the healing process.

Both of these paths (the ascetic and the sensual) teach needed skills to the interested student, but, of the two, movement (especially dance) would seem to be the older and more universal of the transformative techniques. While Eastern meditations are fine for the dedicated student in a religious order, dance, in which the body is given freedom to move as it chooses, is open to everyone, no matter what their level of training. Its effects can be equally strong and life-transforming as the more accepted meditative schools of the East.

When I speak of "dance" here, I am not referring to modern, complicated, choreographed dance. Choreography in which certain complex steps are performed to certain music in a certain way can teach the conscious mind concentration, but it does not offer the mind and body the ecstatic release that comes through the trance dance experience.

Some cultures use choreographed dance figures as a way of moving energy for magical purposes, but they are using concentration, not trance, to achieve their goals. This is why complex choreography works for that kind of magic, but not for the trance that my seasonal ceremonies aim to achieve.

One way to achieve the release of trance dancing is by simple, repetitious movements that, once learned, require no conscious thought. Another way is for the body to be allowed to choose its own movement patterns to the music. In short, the body, not the mind, must direct the activity.

Any simple repetitious motion, repeated again and again to a simple rhythmic beat, can, in time, produce a light trance state. The movements achieve trance by frustrating the conscious mind's need to be always in control. The end result is similar to that obtained by the Eastern meditator; it is merely a different approach to the problem of achieving transformation.

In my ceremonies, we dance non-stop from four to sixteen hours, depending on the length of the entire ceremonial event. If someone tells me they're bored after the first hour, I say to them, "That's very good. That's exactly how you should feel. Now come back to me in another four hours and tell me what you have learned from the experience."

When most modern people hear me talk about dancing all night or all day, they panic, setting up all kinds of mental blocks around the ordeal. Though the ceremony may last for many hours, that doesn't mean that you, personally, have to be on your feet all that time. People can follow their own bodily rhythms, resting as they need to. What it does mean is that you are "present" within the sacred Circle for the whole time, lending your focus and energy to the ritual in some way. What it does not mean is that you are sleeping in some corner for a few hours while others dance. Part of the ceremony is testing yourself a little, by sacrificing your comfort to maintain the integrity of the ritual Circle. As a dancer, drummer, singer, or witness, your presence is important to the well-being and success of the ceremony.

This is as good a point as any to mention breaks. I usually don't schedule any, preferring dancers to follow their own bodily rhythms, with snacks and drinks always available. This also applies to the Dance itself. No one is expected to be on their feet throughout the night; what is expected is that you maintain your energy within the Dance – no crawling off in a corner to sleep for a couple of hours. Your Dance is your spiritual Give-away, your gift to the ancestors and the Gods. It is designed not to be easy.

In the form of the Long Dance ceremonial that I was taught, we use two outer circles of dancers surrounding the inner circle in which the drummers sit, and in which the free-movement trance dancing later occurs. Elizabeth Cogburn calls these two outer rings the yang and yin circles. I have borrowed from her work by continuing to use these names. See Figures 2 and 3, in Chapter 3, for diagrams of all the circles.

The yang ring is the outer circle. Its essence is of air and fire. It is our protection, representing the male aspects of the self. The yang dance is the first step into trance, and the last step as we come out. The movements of this dance are simple, rhythmic, vertical motions. Dancers often carry rattles and stamp out a hard, pounding rhythm in time to the drums. The yang line proceeds in a clockwise circle around the dance ground, creating a ring of fiery protective energy around us.

The movements of the yang line offer grounding and structure, and contain the spiritual energies of the ceremony. At times, when things have gone awry (e.g., the drummers start a jam session from Hell), I have watched dancers instinctively return to the yang line in an attempt to ground and contain the chaos. It is important that this outermost circle, as well as the next circle that is the yin line, be maintained through the whole dance.

If you need to take a break and you are currently dancing on the yin line, move to the yang line for a time before leaving the dance, and start your dance on the yang line again when you come back. When entering or leaving the sacred space of the innermost circle (after it has been opened for the trance dancing), dancers should be certain always to begin and end on the yang line, following the progression yang, yin, inner circle, yin, yang.

The yin ring is the next circle of the dance. Its essence is of water and earth. It represents the softer, female side of the self. Yin is the second step into trance. It is a letting-go of the conscious mind's need to control reality, and an opening and receptivity to the things of the spirit realm. The steps of this dance are simple, flowing, wave-like, side-to-side movements. The instruments of this ring are bells or finger cymbals. The yin ring proceeds counter-clockwise, thus combining with the clockwise yang line to create a sort of gyro effect in the energy patterns of the ceremony.

The movements of the yin line are focused on the pelvis and spinal column. These movements help raise energy from the sexual centres and open the dancer to the inspiration of the Divine. As with the yang line, it is important that this circle be maintained throughout the night. The balance of the sacred energies depends on it.

From the yin line, a dancer, when the time is right, will proceed to the inner circle to dance, in light trance, his or her own dance. I call the innermost circle's movements the "trance dance," although, in fact, dancers should be in trance long before they move into the inner circle. I prolong the dancers' experience on the two outer circles because I have found that this deepens the effect of the free-movement trance dance when it comes, by building up the energy to a greater height.

If dancers proceed into the inner circle too quickly, before the trance state is achieved, what they do is like a stage performance rather than a spiritual inner working. The conscious mind, rather than the teacher within, is doing the work. Going too early to the inner circle means that people tire quickly, then spend the next few hours sitting on the sidelines resting, leaving the dance floor deserted. The point here is balance, learning how to pace yourself and conserve your energies to last out a long night, for at all times some dancers and drummers must be active on the dance ground, to maintain the energy flow.

The movements of the dancers within the inner circle can be very active and manic, or very slow and graceful. Sometimes a dancer may appear to be standing still, but intramuscularly there may be a lot going on. All this is part of the trance experience, which is different for everyone. The effects of the ceremony often go on for months after the dance is over.

We have experimented with how and when to open the inner circle to the trance dance experience. At times, the clan elders or mythical masked figures have danced in the inner circle, inviting other dancers to join them. Perhaps the easiest way, however, is to begin the dance with the drums in the North-East quarter of the inner circle (see the diagrams in Chapter 3), then later retire them to a place by the East Altar outside the circle. (If there is one big drum, the hand-drums take over the beat while the big drum is being moved.) This allows the inner circle to be used in its fullness for the trance dancing.

When I was taught the Long Dance, my teacher Elizabeth allowed free access to the inner space once it had been opened. This often led to congestion in the inner circle, with a neglect of the stabilizing influence of the two outer circles.

I believe this problem arises from the fact that most people in modern society don't know how to distinguish between true trance dancing and "boogy-down" party-time dancing. The difference between the two is not in the movements of the dance, but in where the direction for the movement comes from. When a dancer's channels to the Sacred are opened, through taking the time to deepen one's trance on the yang and yin lines, the body moves very differently than when it is consciously directed.

One of the ways to get around some of this party-time energy is to introduce the following system. When dancers feel they are ready to experience their trance dance, they move to one of the four cardinal points of the inner circle, just inside the yin line. There, one of the West Clan dream-keepers places on their heads a dream hat, that, like the hats worn by some Native spirit dancers, has fringe that covers the face. The dancers are then escorted into the inner space and allowed to dance. They are watched carefully by the dream-keepers, so that no one is injured by bumping into another dancer. This method limits the number of dancers in the inner circle at any one time, since the dream-keepers will admit no one unless there is room, and helps deepen the trance experience for all.

The old people say, "Never dance for yourself alone, but dance for the people too." In traditional cultures, there is far more emphasis placed on service to the community rather than on the psychotherapy aspects of the ritual process. I try to encourage a balance between the two views. As dancers, we are expected to give to, and to draw from, the group energy field. Our dance is our own inner process, and should never be used as a display for the entertainment or admiration (or envy, either) of others. The Dance should be seen as a serious communication with the Sacred Ones we honor.

I guess it is impossible to leave this subject without some discussion of possession. In many cultures around the world, spirit possession, in which the individual's ego blacks out and allows the body to be used by the divine power, is encouraged. In such altered states, people have been known to do amazing feats of healing and other phenomena (such as divination) that would not be possible for them in their normal state of awareness. This type of work is not for the untrained student. Such altered states should only be attempted under the guidance of experienced elders. Never try this on your own, because it can be dangerous.

The seasonal ceremonials I perform do not teach or encourage possession. We work only with the light trance state, and encourage dancers to go only as far out as they can come back unaided. On the rare occasions when someone does get into trouble (crying, screaming or throwing themselves around, or in some way out of control and unable to help themselves), there are experienced people to help out, but rescue work is not viewed with favor, because it drains energy away from the ritual to help the one in trouble.

Doug Morgan, in his book *TTT,* Gabriel Roth, and other modern therapists have come to recognize the part dance and body movement can play in healing. I applaud their work, because it takes the old teachings of indigenous peoples and adapts them to meet the needs of our modern society. Their work is an example of what can be done when the old and the new ways learn to communicate and join forces.

GUIDED VISUALIZATION and Storytelling

A guided visualization is a psycho-spiritual technique in which a narrator takes a relaxed individual (or group of individuals) on an imaginary mental journey. The purpose of this experience is to transform some aspect of the person's life. (For example, to stop smoking, to lose weight, or to begin to feel good about oneself.) The narrator can be there in person or as a disembodied digital voice. The mental imagery combined with a relaxed, open state enables a person to achieve guidance from outside the conscious self, so as to create new patterns of behavior that will be of benefit in all areas of life.

There have been several good books written on the subject of guided visualizations, so I don't propose to re-invent the wheel by re-telling their work here. I would only like to offer a few suggestions from my own experience to add to the knowledge of this craft.

The usual way of leading a guided visualization is to have the audience sit or lie comfortably while the narrator tells or reads them the text of their journey. When I do a visualization, on the other hand, I ask my students to get up and move with the story as it unfolds. (My guided visualizations usually end up as long, story-like affairs.) My reasoning in this is that, if the body is allowed to move with the imagery that the mind is creating, it frees up old traumas stored in the muscular tissues, which can speed the healing process.

I don't mean that a person has to act out every action that is going on in the mind; even a gentle, rhythmic swaying will create the same freeing effect, with less risk of bumping into things or other people. It is the movement, any movement, that seems to be able to bring the changes out of just the mental realm and into a physical reality.

I began using this technique after a workshop of Starhawk's that I attended several years ago. Starhawk does a lot of guided visualizations in her teachings, and I talked to her about how frustrated I felt about them, because as a visually-impaired person I don't "visualize," that is, I don't think or dream in visual images. I told her that I wanted to move around as she talked, not just sit there and be bored.

In the next piece of visualization work we did that week, she invited anyone who wanted to do so to get up and move to the words of her story. I and several others did get up, and it was a whole new experience. For those unable to form clear mental images, for whatever reason, movement is a way around this problem. Since that time, Starhawk has continued to use this technique from time to time, and I know I sure have.

Like Starhawk and a few others, I also use drumming and chants during my work. I use the drum as a rhythmic background drone that helps the body relax and become more open and accessible to the words being spoken. I also use tones, sounds, and vocalized wordless chants as a part of my guided visualizations.

In recent years where it is impractical for participants to move around the space I bring with me a basket of blindfolds which I ask the participants to put on before I begin. I've been told this has a very freeing effect. With everyone blind, no one has to worry about how they look to other people in the room. The participant can totally focus on the inner process and forget about how they might look to others.

I use visualizations many times during a long ceremony, and also as a part of the exercises to prepare for that ceremony. In shorter rituals, the guided visualization is often the main body of work performed by the group.

Both the teller and the participants need to go into light trance to have a successful experience. Those who choose to do this technique need to practise and gain skill, because there is nothing worse than a monotonous voice droning on and on without inflection and style. Such a voice is all too apt to put the listeners to sleep, which is always a danger during the usual guided visualizations anyway, since the participants are sitting or lying in a comfortable position letting their conscious minds drift away.

Another point is the value of learning things by heart, by as much repetition as necessary. This means that you always have them ready for use, as opposed to writing them down, where the paper becomes your memory, and you only remember (if you're lucky) where to find the particular memory you want. It's not necessary to memorize a story or a visualization word-for-word, unless you want to do it that way. All that is needed is to remember the important points of the story, so that you can elaborate them while you tell the story, and not need to read it aloud. A told story is far more impressive, and therefore more significant, to the listener than is a read-aloud one.

A friend of mine says that as an occasional storyteller, she feels embarrassed if she tells a story to an audience that has already heard it. This is totally different from what a traditional storyteller would feel, and shows our eagerness for novelty and our impatience with repetition—and repetition is what makes it possible for us to learn myths and teaching stories well enough to tell them ourselves.

My story-telling technique is very similar to the way I do guided visualizations. I invite the listeners to relax and imagine the tale as it unfolds. I have a drummer to play background sound. I dress in costume, and I chant or tone at various parts of the story. I often walk around as I speak, not for the sake of a dramatic performance, but only as a means of keeping myself in light trance while I am telling the tale. The audience may watch me, or they may close their eyes and drift to where the story takes them; it doesn't matter to me.

Every seasonal ceremony should have a guiding myth, so part of the ritual time should be given over to telling this story to the participants. There may be an existing myth that fits with the ceremony you have planned, but if you cannot find one that works for you, allow yourself to go into trance and create one.

⟡⟡⟡

THE CONE OF POWER

The cone of power is mentioned in several modern books on Wiccan ritual and magic. It is viewed as a powerful technique. It is a way of raising energy with the voice, focusing it, and then releasing it with conscious intent. It is called a "cone of power" because all the energy is focused into a single point above the circle, and thus the lines of energy rising from each participant to the central point outline a cone.

It is done at the time when everyone has been singing and dancing for a while and the energy is high and still building; then, they begin to make sounds or tones with their voices. The volume, and usually the pitch, build and build, until, at just the right moment, the sound rises to a shout that can shake the masonry, or bring mighty heroes trembling to their knees. This is what happens when a cone of power is done right; making noise, however, is not the same as being able to direct the energy of the will through that noise. If it's not done right, therefore, all that happens is that everybody screams, and they all fall to the floor to catch their breath.

I believe this technique is best used in small groups and short rituals with a clear purpose. In large group ceremonials, it often falls flat, so I seldom use it in that context. A small group may be more able to produce a powerful sound than a large one if they have been working together for a good while, and so are more trusting and intimate with each other than a large group is likely to be. Unless your group has had training in martial arts or other voice techniques, the chances are that they will not know how to effectively use their voices to produce a forceful sound. If this is the case for your group, then hold off on the cone until you have the training.

⁂

TALKING-STICK CIRCLES

I use the techniques of the talking-stick circle for my Opening and Closing Councils, but I am describing these circles here because many groups use them as the primary focus of their rituals. Many people believe that this type of circle originated in Native spiritual traditions, but it is used widely today in addiction support groups as well.

How the talking-stick circles work is like this. An object, usually a special stick or a feather, is passed from hand to hand around the circle. The person holding the object has the right to speak, without interruption, while he or she has that object. It can be anything—for instance, a carved stick or staff, an eagle feather, a rock, or a bowl of salt and water. (Just a note about using a bowl, because of its symbolic shape, I use this method a lot with women's groups, but it is an excellent way to teach and maintain focus in any circle. If a speaker gets too carried away they will end up with a wet lap.) The object helps both the speaker and the listeners focus on what is going on. It is a way of respecting each person's opinion and avoiding arguments and talking out of one's turn.

Some groups call talking-stick circles "healing circles" or "healing ceremonies." They can be very moving and powerful to those who attend them. To do these circles well, trust and confidentiality need to be established, because otherwise some people may not feel very confident about opening themselves up. For this reason (i.e., the trust and confidentiality issues), I believe talking-stick circles are best suited to smaller groups that meet regularly, rather than large, open groups of loose affiliations that gather only infrequently.

For many in the New Age, this type of circle is what spirituality is all about. This meets their needs, and they explore no further. In my ceremonies, we use the talking-stick circle in a modified form at our Opening and Closing Councils, and at meetings of the clans within the rituals, but there is so much else going on that it is not a big part of the work.

On the other hand, when I teach small groups or run classes I use this technique a lot. It helps everyone to get to know each other and begin to work together as a group on issues that matter to us all. The core group also uses a talking-stick circle during some of their planning meetings for the seasonal rituals.

There are two points I'd like to make about circles, especially talking-stick circles. First (this one doesn't usually seem to be a problem), a circle is connected. Second, it's round. This means that everyone in a circle that is a circle can see everyone else. An oval is all right too, but the rectangles and squares and kidney-shapes that many groups are prone to just don't work. A friend of mine tells me that she was in one bulge of a kidney-shaped talking-stick "circle" once, and almost half of the participants were out of her sight. She found it extremely difficult to concentrate on what those invisible people were saying, and much of the time she couldn't even hear them well. If you have too many people present for all to hear in a large circle—especially an outdoor circle, then have a smaller circle two rows deep.

⚬✵⚬

THE GIVE-AWAY CEREMONY

The give-away, or potlatch, is a traditional Native American ceremony. As its name implies, the purpose of the ritual is to give away gifts. In the Native community, this ceremony is held as a thanksgiving, as a way of honoring a person (living or dead), or as a way of asking for help with a problem or a healing. An individual or a family can sponsor a give-away, and sometimes they are huge affairs taking months to prepare for, and with thousands of dollars' worth of gifts given by the hosts to the invited guests. This type of ritual expresses the feelings of love and sharing that are so much a part of traditional Native life.

For non-Natives, this is not always an easy concept to understand, but during the long rituals that I am describing there is a similar ceremony that is an adaptation of these older rites. In this newer style, the essence of thankfulness and sharing is preserved, but the preparation is different.

When participants come to these ceremonies, they are asked to bring with them a gift (not wrapped), of spiritual significance to them. The gifts are placed together on a table. When it is time for the give-away ceremony to begin, they are brought to the centre and laid on a blanket. The gifts are then smudged, to relieve them of any negative feelings or any remaining personal energies of their previous owners.

Everyone stands around the blanket in a circle. Usually we sing as the ceremony progresses. We begin with the eldest person present taking the talking-stick and going forward to choose a gift from the blanket. When the gift is chosen, the elder holds up the object for all to see. The person who brought that gift then comes forward and explains a little about why that special thing was chosen, so its new owner will know its history. That person then takes the talking-stick from the elder and continues on with the process of choosing a gift, until everyone has had a turn and all the gifts are claimed.

The give-away can be used in either this modification or the traditional Native form, where all gifts are given by the hosts of the ceremony. I have both given and received gifts of great monetary value in this way, but the purpose is not to show off what you can afford; it is the thought of love and thankfulness that counts. To be able to give an object that means a great deal to you is a gift to the Gods of great value and personal sacrifice.

When I feel I am getting too attached to material things, I know it is time to free up the energy by passing things on in a give-away. Many people cling to their material things, fearing they will go without if they are generous. It doesn't work that way, believe me. If you can see the material world as other forms of energy, and trust in your guides to always take care of you, you will never go without. Only when you think you have to do it all alone, and cling in fear to your things, does want haunt your footsteps.

At a give-away ceremony, your gift can be viewed as a physical symbol of your willingness to give and receive, from spirit as well as from humankind. For this reason, it is important to take some time and care in the selection of the gift you bring.

NOTE: SACRED THEATRE and sacred clowning are a part, and a very important part, of the body of the ritual, but they are discussed at length later, so I am not going to describe them here.

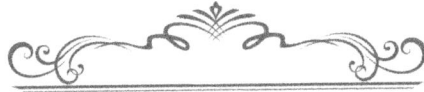

Chapter 7

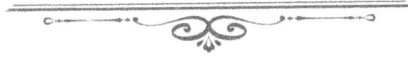

Step 7:
The Conclusion of the Ritual

Releasing the Circle

The Sacred Circle is freed by thanking and releasing each guardian of the directions, and each deity who was invoked when the Circle was cast. This is variously called "opening," "closing," "releasing," or "ending" the Circle.

The closing, including the release of the deities and the guardians of the four quarters, is a part of a ceremony that is often neglected or forgotten, especially by beginners. Picture a typical modern ritual. The main body of the rite is over; it was good and everyone wants to relax. People start talking, refreshments are served, and everyone gets comfortable. Time goes by and people have to leave; they need to go to work early tomorrow, or the babysitter has to go home. For whatever reason, they go. The next thing you know, half the company has left, and the ceremony was never formally concluded and the divine witnesses dismissed. At that point, there may be a hurried attempt to say goodbye to the Sacred Ones and open the Circle, but what about all the people who have already left and are still walking around between the worlds (figuratively speaking)?

It's an old, tried-and-true maxim: If you open a door, you always need to close it again. When you cast the Circle and define sacred space, you step into an altered reality, no matter whether or not it feels any different at the time. A part of your psycho-spiritual being is opened and receptive to outside spiritual influences. Within the Sacred Circle, you are protected, and the influence and guidance you receive should be for your own greater good (assuming you are doing things right). If, however, you leave that Circle casually or in emotional turmoil, without making a formal closure to the rite, then you are leaving yourself wide open for any unseen influence you may come across out there on the street. This includes the psychic influence of other people, as well as of spirits who may or may not be benevolent and well-disposed toward you. Is it any wonder that some people seem to get more anxious and unbalanced after practicing the "old" new religion for a while, rather than becoming healthier? If you know someone like this, check out how loose they are with magical rules.

As for the Goddesses, Gods, and guardians left hanging around, well, at best it's very rude. Put yourself in their place. Would you come back to visit people who called you over and then left and ignored you, without saying goodbye or thanking you? Like so much else, it boils down to a question of respect, for yourself and for others.

Unfortunately, there have been ceremonies that I led where, unknown to me, dancers have left very upset before the event was over. These people had started to process old traumas and became frightened. Instead of talking to someone first, they just left. This happened twice, and I was very worried about those people both times. A high emotional state is not a good reason to leave a ceremony. While still under the protection of the Sacred Circle, try to get help. Perhaps it may not be possible or appropriate to get it from other participants, but at least sit quiet and pray. The Gods are never too busy for rescue work; if you ask, they can help, but don't just leave. Believe me, if you do, you will suffer more than if you stay to work it out.

If for some reason you ever do have to leave a ceremony before the formal closing, always go around and say your own goodbyes to the guardians and deities protecting the space. Make your personal closure yourself, so that when you leave you are grounded and ready to face the outside world.

If you feel troubled by an old ritual that you never let go of, then do the same thing in your mind. Go back to the place and time, see it as clearly as you can, and mentally bid farewell to all those who were there at the time. This will help you make an end to that troubling time in your life. Envision yourself walking out and firmly closing the door behind you after your farewells.

I usually try to save the feast or refreshments until after the formal ending of a ceremony; that way, no one forgets and wanders off before things are concluded. Many New Age chants have been developed to invoke the deities and cast the Circle, but few to release them. Over the years, I have tried to develop chants that close rituals as well as opening them. I believe this part of a ritual is as important as the beginning. At longer rituals, sometimes I ask the clans to design a farewell to the guardians of the directions, rather than a greeting. At first, participants are surprised at this request, but it usually gives them a different perspective on the work.

Just a final word about the direction we take to release the Powers from the Circle. If the Circle was cast in a clockwise direction, then the usual way to open it and release the energy is to go back around it counter-clockwise. Many people share the belief that counter-clockwise is evil and clockwise is good. It's not quite so black-and-white, however. What I was taught is that clockwise movement follows the Sun, and so draws upon the energies that are compatible with the Sun. Counter-clockwise, on the other hand, follows the direction in which the Earth moves. So, if you cast a Circle this way, you are drawing upon the energies that are compatible with the Earth rather than on Solar power.

To work evil, many bad shamans or magicians choose to use Earth energy, because of its connection with the Underworld, but in itself the counter-clockwise direction is neither bad nor good. Besides, below the equator the whole thing changes anyway.

Some women's groups are choosing to do their rituals in a counter-clockwise manner, not because they wish to work evil, but because of its connection with the Earth and female power. When I go into the Underworld, I always cast the Circle counter-clockwise and open it clockwise. (This would generally be a second Circle, within the larger Circle that was cast clockwise for the ritual as a whole.) These counter-clockwise Circles are just a few more examples of how we can create symbol systems that work for us, rather than rule us.

Remember that, in addition to releasing the deities and opening the Circle, you need to ground the excess energy remaining within yourself back into the Earth. (This does not mean draining yourself to exhaustion; it simply means that if you took up more energy than you yourself needed for the ceremony, you must release the excess.) If you do not, you are likely to feel drunk or spacey, and not all there, and it is not wise for you to try to drive a car or do other mundane things until you have grounded the energy and come back to the present. The simplest way to do this is to bend down, place your palms on the Earth, and imagine the energy draining out of you. It is also possible to ground yourself with deep breathing, and eating is very grounding as well, which is another reason I recommend serving food at the end of a ceremony.

THE CLOSING COUNCIL

At our longer community rituals, we usually end with a Closing Council. During this time, the talking stick (or other object) is passed around, and participants are given a chance to speak about their experience during the rite. (I described talking-stick circles at greater length in Chapter 6.)

With a large group, it is usually not possible to give each person unlimited time to speak, but most people have more to share at this time than they did at the Opening Council. As a rule of thumb, I allot each person at most five minutes to speak. As with the Opening Council, we use a series of questions to help structure the participants' responses. These include such things as "What did you receive from the ceremony? What was hard for you, and how did you deal with it? What were some of your favorite moments during the event?" These questions help participants to focus on saying the most in the shortest amount of time.

Bear in mind that the ritual is not completely over when you finally leave the site. Like dropping a pebble into a pond, the ripples will be felt for long afterward, in other areas of your life. Many people don't realize that as long as two or three years later, they may still be processing something that came up for them during a particular ceremony. This is a perfectly natural process, which is quite different from what may happen if you go away from a ritual without closing the Circle first. You handle the processing in a more balanced manner, because if you don't do the closure you are more open and vulnerable.

To avoid stress and unbalance, a good and thorough grounding should always be done, both at the beginning and at the end of a rite, but be aware that the spiritual work you have done will take time to mature. In our modern schools, we are taught to view events and lessons as separate or linear, when in fact things are far more connected than may be apparent at first.

At this point in our history these seasonal ceremonials are often a new and sometimes a very profound experience for people attending the rite. Inner "stuff" that gets brought up during the ritual may take months or even years to fully understand and integrate into our lives. Some participants will go home to family and friends who won't understand what they have experienced. For these people, the ceremony, in hindsight, can be a very isolating and depressing experience if there is no one around to talk to and to share what is going on for them.

For this reason, it is wise, when planning the ritual, to set up a support system or network for afterwards, so that dancers can speak to someone about their experiences and the emotions they are processing. Logically, the clan elders should fill this role, but there could be another member of the clan who does this, especially if the elder is a little tired from planning and participating in the ritual just completed.

The next step, of course, is to set up stable clan groups that meet on an ongoing basis. In time, these groups can become very close, and do much of the spiritual work together that is so much a part of the preparations for the large seasonal ceremony.

Eventually, I would hope that a system like that of the Pueblo Indians of the Southwest can develop, in which each clan takes responsibility for sponsoring one of the major seasonal rites. This system has worked for thousands of years for them, and can for others as well. Right now, for most groups, that isn't practical, because the stable numbers willing to participate are not there yet. For this reason, the same group, with minor changes, may be responsible for organizing rite after rite. It is therefore important to prevent burnout for as long as possible.

In general, when I have experienced burnout, it has been because I have invested too much of my own vital energies in a project, rather than allowing myself to be guided by Spirit, and trusting that what I can't do, Spirit will find someone else to do, if it truly needs to be done.

Burnout can also occur when clear duties and boundaries aren't set up ahead of time. This means that some members, who have underlying "need to be in control issues that enable them to feel safe, take on more than they are physically able to accomplish, while others drift around, looking for work. This is where core group meetings after the event are equally as important as before the rite. In these later meetings, members can analyze what worked and what didn't, and how to do better next time. It is also important to keep the communication flowing within the group, so that if personal conflicts arise, they can be dealt with without being left to fester or be gossiped about later. Two people talking about a third, not present, and other forms of gossip, can be so damaging, and so easily done, with no malice intended. Great effort is needed to keep gossip and miscommunication from destroying the delicate fabric of our ritual system.

⚭

THE CLEANING-UP AND Storing-away

After a long ceremony with little sleep, the last thing anyone wants to think about right away is clean-up. Some may prefer to return after a few hours sleep to tackle the job, but I prefer to do as much as possible at the time and be done with it. Waiting till later may mean that some of the potential work crew has gone off to home and elsewhere, and so there may be fewer people available to do the work.

It is the main responsibility of the East, South, and West clans to take charge of the general clean-up. (The North clan took care of registration and served the food, so they have less responsibility for clean-up.) This means the whole clans, not just the clan leaders; their sole responsibility is taking down their altars. As part of the teachings of honor and respect, the ritual site should be left as clean, or cleaner, than the way it was found. This will guarantee your welcome back should you ever wish to use the site again, and shows respect for other people (the owners or caretakers of the place) and for the land.

Sometimes it is hard to ensure that clan members will stay to help. Community spirit and responsibility are often talked about, but not so often accomplished. I usually talk about this during the Opening Council and encourage dancers to make a commitment to help afterwards as part of their ceremonial pledge, but it may take time for that message to sink in. People are so used to having things done for them that it's hard to get over that block.

A handy trick I learned from some Seattle Pagans I know is to charge everyone an extra five dollars at the beginning of the rite. Those who stay to clean up split the money collected. If everyone stays, then they all break even and the work is quickly done; if only one or two people stay, they go home with a large chunk of money, and so don't feel taken advantage of. It works like a charm, though I hope in time a group that worships together often will get past such necessary incentives.

As in the set-up, only the clan leaders should be responsible for packing up their shrines. Your group will have to decide if there is a central place to store all the clan gear, or if the clan leaders will each keep their own altar furnishings at their homes. If the altar things are to be held in a central place, I suggest the Dragon Clan leader take on the role of protector, to keep the items till the next ceremonial.

If you plan to do a number of ceremonies with the same core people, I would suggest having your clan leaders hold the same office for at least a full year before passing it on. A person can spend a lifetime deepening into the craft, and still never become close to knowing it all, but a year is at least a step on the path. During that time, these leaders will have a chance to go so much deeper with their craft. They can really get to know the totem animals of their direction, and the deeper feelings and meanings of the power of their elements.

After everything is clean, I usually go back over it and smudge the site, just to break up and renew the energies of the area. In a publicly-used place, our residual energy patterns may be just as upsetting to the next users of the site as the old energies of earlier occupants were to us, so as a final gesture of consideration, I like to leave the area in a neutral state.

A last thought about cleansing and storing the ritual tools: If there has been a lot of emotional work done at a rite, or in general as a precaution, I like to cleanse my things before I put them away for their final rest until the next time they are needed. There are several types of cleanses I know of, and I use one or more at a time.

Using the element of Air, items can be smudged, and I usually do that right on the site before I bring them home, regardless of whether I do any other cleansing of them as well. There is also a Fire cleansing, in which non-flammable items are passed through a flame. In keeping with both the Air and Fire energy, ritual items may be left outside in a safe place in the wind and sun for a few days.

The most common way I know next is to cleanse items with the element of Water. (Naturally, this form is to be used only with things that will not be damaged by water!) Wash or soak the items in a solution of salt and water, or just clear spring water. (Adding the salt brings Earth into the cleanse along with Water.) Tied down in some way, tools may also be left in a fast-running creek for a time, which allows the swift water to carry downstream any unwanted emanations, though I would suggest keeping an eye on your tools if you do this, so they don't float away along with the unwanted energies. The water diffuses and breaks up existing energy patterns, so they won't cause any harm downstream.

Lastly, if something feels really heavy or icky, you need to bury it in the Earth for a while. The Earth's grounding neutral energy will do the job, if anything can. Remember to mark the spot where you have buried it, of course. I often just set my tools or crystals right on the Earth, where they can be exposed to sun, wind, earth, and possibly rain energy. Especially if I have been asked to work at a healing where a lot of old traumas have come up, I will do this even before I take anything into the house, because I don't want to bring a residue of that stuff in to affect myself or my family later.

Many people in the healing professions don't take enough care of themselves and their space. They don't always cleanse or change their energy fields from one client to the next. When this happens, everyone holds on to each other's negativity, and it is passed back and forth from one treatment to the next. Women, especially, feel that they have to take on the pain of the world, and once they have done so, they don't know how to ground and release it.

After cleansing and storing away my gear, I take a bath with herbs, or baking soda and Epsom salts, and change my clothes. All these fine details are a part of the process too, that need to be remembered to ensure a safe ritual practice.

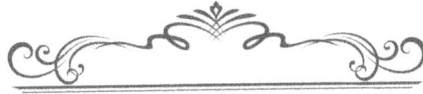

Chapter 8

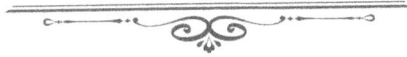

Ritual Rules of Thumb

Every group that comes together to perform ritual needs to work within some basic set of rules. Rules may vary from group to group or from ritual to ritual, but some sort of guidelines should be established, so that everyone knows what to expect of themselves and those around them. The suggestions I make here are ones I have found through trial and error to work the best for large group ceremonies. I offer them merely as recommendations, not as absolute truths.

TARDINESS AND IDLE Chatter

If someone has made a commitment to take part in a ceremony and the time has been agreed on by the group, everyone should make a point of being on time. For those who are chronically late, this may present some problems. However, except for emergencies, lateness reflects a lack of respect for the self, for the rite, and for those who have gathered to perform it.

When people hang around chatting, waiting for a few late members to arrive, the energy gathered and focused on performing the ritual is drained away. How many times have I watched people gathered for a ceremony hang around for a half an hour or more, idly talking about who broke up with whom, and what was coming up on TV tomorrow night, while their energies wind down to the point that, when they finally begin, little power is left for the rite.

If you have to wait for a rite to begin, spend the time constructively in meditation and prayer, rather than socializing. I've known of groups who waste their entire time together talking, only realizing too late that the time is over and other obligations call, and so no rite can be performed. I suggest socializing after the ritual, over tea and cake or a feast, rather than before the event.

It's natural to want to talk to the people you circle with, but your group needs to decide what its priorities are – ritual or socialization. Some groups solve this problem by meeting twice a month: once for ritual, once for a party. This is often a good compromise, because through the social events trust can be strengthened between members of the group.

It goes without saying that, if you are responsible for setting up the site, you should allow enough time to do that, so that no one has to wait around for all the preparations to be completed. Unless creating the space is a part of the ritual itself and all members of the group participate, waiting around for its completion is equally as draining as waiting for people to arrive.

The question of allowing late-comers into a ritual that has already begun is an individual decision of each group. As a general rule, I would recommend that, after the Circle is cast, no one be allowed in. Late-comers usually feel disoriented and out of step with what is happening when they join a ritual-in-progress, and their presence can throw off the balance of the energies you are trying to contact as well. Taking a laid-back attitude is quite common, but if the intent of the rite is more than just a social one, then it can be dangerous to mess around with the energies that have been invoked by passing in and out of a Circle when members arrive late.

If a group decides it will allow late-comers to enter a ritual, it should be made clear that it is the responsibility of those late-comers to take the time to ground themselves, and clear their minds and spirits of whatever it was that made them late, before they enter the Circle. This is necessary because many people are very sensitive to turmoil in others, and if you are late because, for instance, you had a fight with your spouse, and you are still rehashing it in your mind when you enter the Circle, your agitation will communicate itself to the rest of the group and damage the ritual. Even if you were late merely because you were trying to finish whatever you were doing before the meeting, you will be in a hurried, scattered condition when you arrive, which will impede your and the group's efforts to achieve a tranquil, meditative state of mind.

DRUGS AND ALCOHOL

When I was being trained in Native ways, one of the first and most strongly-enforced rules I learned was no drugs or alcohol at a ceremony. There are a lot of reasons for this strictness; some of them are cultural, some spiritual in nature. I will explain the spiritual reasons later in this section, but the cultural reasons have to do with the devastation that alcohol has caused to Natives and Native culture.

Now that I use European rituals a lot, I sometimes pass a cup of wine (or juice) as part of my rites, but I use alcohol only as a sacrament, never as a means of getting high, either before or during a ritual. Getting high at ceremonies, to me, is a very risky and dangerous business, because I learned in my Native training that it invites possession, or at least an increased openness to negative influences.

Many people use alcohol or drugs as an important part of their rites, because they feel it increases their receptivity and opens them up to the Gods. I agree that it increases your receptivity, but you have no control over what you receive when you are stoned, and you may not like what you get. Also, it is a crutch, and if you depend on drugs and alcohol to enter ritual space, you will never learn to progress beyond a certain point, or be able to achieve magical power without artificial help.

If you can view a ritual as a living being, then having people get high is like having a diseased organ within the body. People's energies are not in control, and are out of balance with each other and the universal powers called to witness the rite.

Spiritually, most Native teachers say that, when you're under the influence of drugs or alcohol, you are very open and very vulnerable to psychic attack. This is another reason why sacred herbs were confined to use within the protective Circle. Every psychic or medicine man I know will agree that, when you are high, your aura is wide open to friend or foe. So why take the chance? If you are afraid or nervous about what will be taking place at a ritual, and feel you need drugs or alcohol to keep your courage up, talk about it instead, or find another way of coping with your concerns. Or, if it's that scary, don't go. You're either not ready, or there is something very wrong at that particular rite.

Some people use a ritual as an excuse for getting stoned. Others use the fact that they are already high as an excuse to have a ritual. It should be pretty clear by now that I feel both practices are extremely unwise. However, I know that there are many who believe that a ceremony ought to be a celebration, and for some people, celebrating means getting high. I believe that the spiritual rules I was taught are good and effective ones, but I remind myself that my ways are not the only ways.

Racially, most Natives have a low tolerance for alcohol. It was not a part of most northern Native cultural experience before contact with Europeans. Since contact, its effects have been devastating. It would be unthinkable for most Natives to consider using wine or mead as a sacred substance, which is still another confusing issue between the races. When they see white Pagans using alcohol in their rituals, it is hard for them to overcome their cultural prejudices and accept that the Pagans are performing a sacred rite according to their own cultural standards.

When drugs were used (such as peyote and magic mushrooms), they were used only under very strict supervision by the elders, and only on sacred occasions. Until recently, it would have been inconceivable to use a sacred herb at certain times for prayer and at other times for recreation. As far as I know, northern Native cultures had no recreational drugs before the Europeans arrived.

When a plant like peyote is used for ritual purposes, it is gathered in a special sacred way, usually by the Elder conducting the ceremony, or by his helpers or apprentices. These plants are treated as holy, and never used outside certain ritual contexts, never for a recreational high (at least not by the old teachers). The Natives who used such sacred plants did not regard them as chemicals that would cause a specific physical or mental effect. Instead, they prayed to the spirits of the plants, and regarded them as teachers who would guide their worshippers on their spiritual paths. This is a whole different energy pattern from buying drugs from the dealer (or the liquor store) down the block, and sometimes using it in a sacred way and sometimes not.

⬥

SEXUAL ENERGY (WHAT to do with it or about it)

During a powerful ritual, sexual energy may be raised, either consciously or by accident. The question is, what to do with that energy when it is aroused? No one should feel unsafe at a community ceremonial because they have been propositioned on the way to or from the washroom, nor should attendance at any ritual be used as an excuse to meet secretly with a lover, undetected by parents or a current partner. These things do happen, but they are due to a mishandling of the energies and to a lack of respect for one's self and for others.

As a guideline, sexual energy that is generated within a ritual context should remain within the sacred Circle. In Elizabeth Cogburn's Long Dance tradition, this would mean dancing the energies out, either with a partner (if you are both strongly attracted to each other) or on your own, as a trance-dance within the inner circle of the dance floor. Sexual energy is best not acted on directly, but transformed and used as a power-source, for the well-being of the whole ceremony and everyone present. Going off to the bushes for a quick one is not the answer, because it takes members and their energy fields out of the Circle and drains the rite.

One difference between Native ceremonies and European rites is that many modern Pagans encourage sexual energy at their rituals. Usually it is only present symbolically, as knife put into cup (symbolizing sexual union of male and female), but I know of cases where group sex rituals do occur. ("All acts of pleasure are my rituals" is often quoted as a maxim of the Goddess.) The danger here is that group and public sex walk a fine line between religious rite and debauchery, in my opinion.

The aim in any ritual should be to keep the energies strong and focused, and the intent clear. If the sexual act, in symbol or fact, will aid in doing that, then, if the question arises, consider it. If it will disrupt the group and have negative repercussions later, or destroy the group harmony, then I would suggest treading very carefully.

⟋⟋⟋⟋⟋

THE PARTICIPATION OF Children

Philosophically speaking, the cult of the child flourishes within the New Age. Childhood is romanticized as being the age of innocence and heightened spirituality. (The Victorians felt the same way about it.) I find this cult fascinating, because it is so different from the Native view that old age is the time to be valued, because of its greater wisdom and spirituality.

I believe there are several reasons for the cult of the child, one being that modern society has a fear of the sexually mature body and therefore idealizes the supposedly non-sexual child, and another is perhaps our unconscious hope that the youth of today will rescue us all from destruction in their innocent wisdom and God-like qualities. (When I hear people talk like this, I wonder if they have ever raised teen-agers.)

Still another reason for the cult of the child, in my opinion, centres around issues of authority. People who felt overly-restricted in their own childhood – and people who indeed were badly over-restricted—may try to live out their fantasies of an idyllic, utterly-free youth by bringing up their own children without rules or structure.

What this worship of the child may mean is that children are given license to attend, and often disrupt, New Age rites, without being disciplined or corrected for their rude behavior. It goes without saying that, if we want to have our new ways carried on to future generations, we need to instruct the young in our teachings. On the other hand, when children are allowed a free hand to disturb the adults, they probably aren't able to learn anything at that time anyway, except perhaps another way to get attention.

Childless people who may be bothered by children's behavior often feel they shouldn't complain about it, because our society already puts tremendous burdens on parents (especially mothers). Thus, well-meaning people without children are reluctant to put a further strain on already-oppressed parents, who may not be able to attend a rite at all if they cannot bring their kids. Also, many childless people know better than to tell anyone else how to bring up their children. I am a mother myself, however, and I can therefore legitimately object to disruptive children without fear of being called a child-hating grinch.

When children are allowed to run in and out or talk and laugh among themselves while sitting in the Circle, then everyone suffers. The ritual itself suffers, because energy that should be focused on the intent of the rite will be drawn away to deal with controlling unwanted behavior. The child suffers, because he is being forced to be present when he may not wish to be (or to stay at a ritual that is not as exciting as he expected), and he may carry away, not the teachings that his care-givers may wish him to receive, but more negative feelings of frustration and rebellion.

The parents or care-givers suffer, because their attention is divided between the ritual and their child, and because they may feel resentful of the child's interruptions, and both guilty about disturbing others and angry at others for being disturbed by the child's perfectly natural behavior. The other adults suffer, because their concentration is broken and they may feel angry and resentful at the interruption.

It is the hope of many parents today that, by sharing with our children our Pagan ways, they will grow up with a new sense of caring for the Earth, and learn to love others and treat them well and with respect. These are noble ideals that are right to have, but if the child is not ready or doesn't want to be there, then it is pointless to insist. The experience will be as negative as forcing children of earlier generations to attend Sunday school (for their own good, of course).

A child may be curious about what the adults around him are doing, but I would advise taking it slow. Give your rites a sense of mystery. Allow short periods where children can witness a part of a ritual, but keep the rest separate. When children willingly want, and have earned the right, to participate in adult ceremonies, the experience will be treated with far more respect, and the child will learn more in one ritual than in a hundred which he has been forced to attend. Some children may want to attend a rite, or think they do, but become bored and restless after a short time. Parents need to judge their own children's attention span, and either insist that a child not come to a rite until he or she is ready to last through all of it, or else make arrangements beforehand to have another care-taker come in to take the child away after a short time.

Parents of young children are often faced with the dilemma that, if they can't bring their children, they can't attend at all. Our modern society is lacking in support for mothers and children, and I know from personal experience the heart-wrenching predicament that parents can face, especially during the early years, when children are too young to be left alone should they be unable or unwilling to come. Groups that have a lot of members with young children should probably consider a group solution to the babysitting problem, rather than leaving it once again as another issue to isolate mothers who wish to participate.

The group may consider a parallel rite (for short rituals, of course), where the children meet in a separate room and the adults take turns supervising the kids. The Sunday Schools of Christian churches do much the same thing. For longer rites, what could be done is to arrange for a paid babysitter for all children of participants who need it, with the babysitter's payment considered as an expense of the rite as a whole, paid for from the general registration fees.

Many of the ceremonies that I conduct are very long, and involve a lot of inner work. For most of the ritual, it would be too distracting to have young children present. Also, it is not fair to them to expect such long periods of concentration and discipline. A guideline I sometimes use is to say that children are welcome to participate if they are old enough to fully accept the discipline that is demanded by the ceremony, or young enough that their care-giver can accept it for them. (In short, over 16 or babies.) If the babies cry, their care-givers should take them outside where they will not disturb the ritual. Because of the needs of babies, their mothers will usually take the role of a witness rather than a full participant, and dance only on the yang line.

There is always the possible exception of the uncommonly well-behaved five-year-old, but especially if there are a group of children present with no planned activity for them to do, and no special place for them to be, they tend to hang around, get bored, and demand attention, which adults then have to see to. This may not be a problem for short, loosely-organized events, but if you are planning a rite lasting long hours or days, with a lot of intense inner work to be done, the distraction and disruption of children present is a drain on the group and the event.

Mothers with infants who are not yet walking have come to the ceremonies I facilitate, but can only participate in limited ways, because the demands of their children keep them from going completely into the experience in the same way that other participants might. Working within these limitations, I find, has a certain discipline that brings great rewards, if the mother can accept those limitations without feeling angry or resentful. I have learned that part of life's challenge is to embrace and utilize the circumstances that we are faced with anyway.

Another suggestion of how to include children and other family members would be to invite them to a portion of the rite, such as a feast, while keeping most parts of the event restricted to participants only. This will let them know a little of what you are doing, and give them something to look forward to when they are older.

Our children are our future, and it is my hope that, with care, we can teach them in such a way that they will want to pass on our new-old Pagan ways to their children and their children's children. My intention in writing this book, all through it, has been to aid in the establishment of new and life-affirming traditions that will last through many centuries to come.

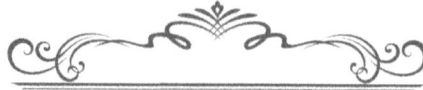

Chapter 9

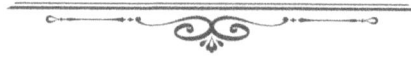

Sacred Theatre

Before we begin this discussion, we should take a moment to describe my perception of what sacred theatre is. First of all, as its name implies, it is theatre which is done within the context of a ritual or seasonal rite lasting several days, rather than for entertainment. Secondly, the performance can be the entire ritual, or only a part of a longer rite. Lastly, whether the enactment is a retelling of old myths, a comedy, a tragedy, a song, or a dance, it is undertaken and performed in the spirit of dedication to the Gods. This attitude of service and offering is what separates this type of performance from mere entertainment.

Theatre began as ritual. Our ancestors, of whatever cultural tradition, used theatre as a means of communication and connection between humanity and the Divine. Many spiritual traditions dedicated both the theatrical performance (the ceremonial) and the actor/priests themselves to the service of the Gods. The first plays were dramatic retellings of ancient myths and stories. They were usually performed as a part of a larger seasonal ceremony. The purpose of these plays was to teach the old ways to the young, and to strengthen the bonds between the human community and the divine forces which watched over them and their world.

When performing, the ancient actor (or modern indigenous one) would dress in costume and mask. These masks were honored and treated with respect, for the mask was like a storage cell of energy for the archetype or deity it represented. The mask had a spirit of its own, and was treated like a living being, including being ceremonially fed from time to time. When the actor put on the mask, his or her personality slid aside so that the spirit of the mask could use the actor's body during the ritual performance.

The actor's craft was a part of the religious training in the past, and still is in places like Bali and India where theatre and religion are still united today. A secularized theatre performed only for entertainment, as we know it in the West, is a fairly modern concept. By the Renaissance, a budding theatre-for-entertainment had been established. During this time, actors began performing bare-faced (without masks), and the purpose of the theatre shifted more and more away from religious instruction to entertainment that would please an audience.

When I took acting classes, I was amazed at how much of the training I received was similar to what I had learned in my spiritual studies. Some of the old spiritual exercises are still there, though disguised from their ancient roots. The modern theatre has, for the most part, forgotten from whence it came.

In a way, this is a great tragedy, because the actor today is still tapping into and channeling much of the old archetypal energy, but without the advantage of the priest or shaman's training to go with it, the modern actor is often unable to cope with those unseen forces unleashed by his art. Once the doors to the cosmos have been opened and the actor is channeling those forces, which all good performers must do, few know how to close down the doors again when the energy is no longer needed.

I believe (my own pet theory) that that is why the incidence of alcohol and drug abuse is so high among theatre folk. They have opened Pandora's Box, and they have never learned how to close down the lid and ground the energies they use. So, to handle the stress, they may resort to what comes easy: drugs and alcohol. I hope that someday this will change, but most actors I have talked to about my pet theory are not very religious, and so are amused or offended by my suggestions.

I also believe that theatre is the missing aspect of most New Age rites. It is time to return theatre to its ancient roots, and bring it back within the power of the sacred Circle. To do this, we need to look at theatre in a different way. The typical modern production is performed on a raised stage with lots of props, costumes, and fancy lighting. The audience sit below, usually entirely passively, expecting to be entertained.

The old theatre was performed within the sacred Circle. There were few props, no fancy lighting effects, and the audience often interacted with the performers. The actor priest/priestesses wore masks and manifested in the rite the power and authority of the Gods. This tradition of the theatre is still very much alive in some Native communities today. I have heard stories of actors speaking through long hollow kelp stems to speak for the spirits, and of others who swim out in the cold ocean waters, breathing underwater through hollow reeds, only to appear in full costume and mask on the beach, just as an old hero or monster would have done in the ancient tales.

SACRED MASKS

I strongly support bringing back the use of the sacred mask to ritual theatre. Sacred masks can be a great responsibility for those who have them in their care. They must be treated with respect, kept safe, not displayed like art objects in your living room, and symbolically given food and water from time to time. In return, these masks act as a storage battery for the power of the Sacred. When the actor puts on the mask, its power will flow into him or her and strengthen the ritual performance.

The next question is, what kind of mask to use? In the older traditions, masks were molded from clay or carved from a large gourd or wood (sometimes from a living tree). In the Orient, sacred masks are often made from papier-mache. If you have skill with wood or clay, you can make a mask from those materials, but a simpler, yet still durable, way is to make a mask using plaster strips molded to the human face. (Cover it with Vaseline first!)

When partially dry, the mask is removed from the actor's face, allowed to dry completely, and finished off. With a little time and skill, you can create real works of art, complete with head-dress and paint. Masks like this are molded to a particular person's face and thus cannot comfortably be worn by other people, so they are not as well suited for handing down from one generation of priests to the next as the old-style wooden masks, but they will last for years and can be as much a home for spirit power as a wooden mask can.

In the past I have had two masks in my care. Both came to me in dreams and their spirits directed me to create them. They are powerful ceremonial objects, and I only brought them out at special times. Those masks were full-face masks. They were great for dancing or just to look upon, but they weren't good if I needed to make long speeches or chant. What we of the modern tradition have forgotten how to do is to speak through a mask loudly and clearly. (Some old masks may have had a megaphone effect in their structure, while others inevitably muffle the voice.) Except for the Greeks, most ancient theatre was mimed, with a narrator telling the story, rather than the masked dancers trying to speak lines.

I would suggest that, if you are creating masks for actors who will have speaking roles, you make half-masks and paint the lower part of the actor's face to match the mask. This will give the feeling of a full-face mask, but allow the actor freedom to speak naturally.

An interesting quality that John Keystone notes in his mask work is the ability of the mask to take on certain personal characteristics, no matter who is the actor wearing it. He cites examples of different classes of his students, who had no knowledge of previous work, exhibiting similar behaviors when the same masks were put on. This is in keeping with what I learned from my Elders, who speak of the mask having a spirit of its own.

An actor in full costume and mask can have a powerful effect on the watchers. In this craft, body movements and tone of voice must convey the meaning, because there is no eye contact or facial expression to help. This type of craft relies most heavily on the actor's skill and the Sacred Power directing him/her to create the desired effect.

Just a further comment here about using animal skins and preserved heads for sacred rites. I have known people who have since childhood had a psychic connection sometimes to an individual animal or to the spirit of a particular group of animals that some Natives and Non-Natives refer to as Totems. These "Totems" are seen as guides and protectors and often appear in some form or other at larger Native events.

Most people I have met in the modern pagan community are too loose with this term and haven't allowed themselves to know these Spirits at a deep level. This is partially the fault of our living in urban areas where you really can't know a wolf or a bear intimately. (Though you may be able to tap into ancestral memories if your familial and racial heritage has such knowledge.) The point here, is to be cautious with the use and the invoking of such beings until you have experience and skill in your spiritual practice to use such power for the good of not only yourself but your community.

Sacred theatre relies on the power of both the actors and the witnesses to creatively re-create reality through imagination. We must be able to believe and accept that our serious play within the sacred Circle can change reality, not only there, but in the outer world as well. This is the gift of the theatre. With all its pageantry, it helps our adult minds to believe and accept as real what we are trying to achieve with our sacred rites.

⚶

IMPROVISATION

The ability to respond to the imagined as if it were real is the cornerstone of both the theatre and magic ritual. Elizabeth Cogburn calls this "serious play with a purpose," and it is a vital skill in the ceremonial art. Most adults have lost this ability, but the next time you can, watch a young child at play; this may help you reclaim the forgotten techniques.

A six-year-old enters totally into the spirit of his or her play. Without embarrassment or inhibitions, children "become" the characters they imagine. Everything in the game becomes so real that an old stick is transformed into a magic sword, while a big pillow by the TV becomes a mighty war horse. Children are natural magic users. In their unskilled hands, this energy is only for play, but the energy is the same that the actor and the Spirit Healer use to recreate reality within the sacred Circle or the theatrical experience.

By the time most of us have reached adulthood, we are unable to imagine and recreate reality in this way. As we grew older, we acquired a lot of inhibitions, till the fear of embarrassment or looking foolish in front of others prevents us from responding totally to the sacred Circle and achieving our ritual goals. With training and practice, many of these unhealthy habits can be overcome. If I have a student who is shy, I recommend that he or she take acting classes to help overcome the nervousness in front of others.

Of all my experiences with the secular theatre, I value my classes in improvisation the most. In improv, there are no set scripts to learn; everything is created on the spot. The actors receive characters or a situation, and they have to come up with plot and dialogue right there, as the interaction of the play progresses. This method of theatre, more than any other, relies on the actors' skill and imagination. Like the ritual experience, the performer of improv must, through his or her imagination, create a situation and respond as if it were real. Once again, this is serious play, but this time without a divine purpose.

When I do invocations or guided visualizations, I never rely on a memorized text; I always improvise what I am saying. I usually start with a general idea of what I will say, and then I relax and allow whatever comes to be channeled through me.

In the old days, many travelling theatre companies, such as the *Commedia del Arte* in Italy, worked this way. Each player had a character that they assumed for years at a time. This other personality became so much a part of them that the interacting dialogue between players was never scripted, but allowed to unfold naturally at each performance. Like modern psycho-dramas in therapy sessions, as well as role-playing games such as Dungeons & Dragons, these early plays were probably very powerful works of art. They bear further exploring by the modern ceremonialist.

I am aware that most New Age ritual is not done with improvisation. Most people either read or memorize their lines for a ceremony. Of the two, memorization is always the way to go, because reading a piece doesn't allow for the free flow of energy during the ritual experience; the conscious mind must always be in control, to focus on the printed text.

To use improvisation effectively, however, a group must be fairly small and close-knit, in order to be able to interact with each other without restraint and in perfect trust. This is certainly a goal to strive for in our communities and covens.

As in older times, I can envision modern groups of travelling players once more moving around to different gatherings and Pagan rites to perform dramas that tell the ancient tales and express the feelings of the people. To do this, groups must come together and work on exploring the possibilities of plot and character development through the tools of improv.

Let me offer an example of a more secular nature, but useful is displaying how a group may use improvisation to develop a sacred drama. A few years ago, I worked with a Native theatre group in my town. We wanted to create a play for an upcoming festival that would reflect the search that many young Natives face in trying to find their roots. There were four of us in the core group working on this project with others lending their support and doing behind the scenes stuff. One of us was a young woman who had been adopted away from her people as a child. Her strongest wish was to go back to her reserve and find her grandmother, and ask her to teach her the old ways. This became our plot.

In the tale, her name was Rose. The first scene showed Rose in her city life, drifting, unhappy, but finally making up her mind to overcome her fear of being rejected and go back to the reserve. The next scene showed the old grandma meeting with Rose on the reserve and agreeing to teach her. The last scene, mostly done in dance, showed Rose going on a vision quest and receiving guidance from a spirit helper.

All in all, there were four people on stage needed for this play: a narrator who gave background information at the beginning of each scene, Rose, her grandmother, and a fourth person who played a friend in the bar in the first scene and Rose's spirit guide (masked) in the last scene.

This play was well received by many audiences, because it touched on some real issues for many young Native people, but the characters were more archetypal in nature than personal, which is also why their appeal was so strong. This was a great experience for me, and one of the first I had of working in this way. I can see its potential for the sacred as well. The same steps I used in creating Rose's play could be followed to recreate the old legends.

The dialogue we created to go with the plot of this story was generated by a combination of improvisation and memorization. Once we had the plot blocked out, what I did was to take everyone through a guided visualization in which I grounded them and brought them to their power places to dip into the well spring of creativity. I had them mentally become the characters they were going to portray. After that, I asked each character in turn to get up and walk back and forth with eyes unfocussed and partly closed. Where there was a dialogue between two characters, they both did this at the same time, so they could create their conversation within their joint meditations. They were to continue walking until the scene fixed in their mind's eye and words started to flow.

At that point, the dialogue was either recorded on tape or written down on paper by other members of the cast. We did this for each character in each scene until everything felt complete. Then we worked on memorizing the lines, or at least key phrases that were another actor's cue lines (leaving some limited room for improvisation during the actual performances).

By involving the body as well as the mind in the creation of a play, one seems to "move" through the process with a power that is not always available to the mind alone. I recommend this exercise anytime a group gets stuck and doesn't know how to proceed in developing a ritual performance. This is a very powerful technique that I use a lot, in developing theatre and in other exercises, such as dancing out a dream rather than talking about it. It is a very true statement that no change is complete until it is manifested in the body. Our bodies are our greatest guides and teachers.

Another exercise that I often do with groups, to help them add depth to their rites and get away from reading a script, is to plan out the moves of a rite (who does what when), and then perform the actual ritual in vocalized sounds, with no identifiable words allowed. This forces the power to be generated by other means entirely than the words we are so accustomed to. It isn't easy, but this method will totally change and deepen your experience of the ritual arts. There isn't time or space to go into much detail here, but I would direct the interested reader to William Pennell Rock's book, *Performing Inside Out*. In this book there is a step-by-step procedure for going through the whole ritual theatre process. I found his work very exciting, and highly recommend it as a must for anyone interested in using sacred theatre.

There is another type of theater I had the good fortune to witness a few years ago that I would like to learn more about because I believe it could have potential for use in healing ceremonies and conflict resolution situations, such as what came up between Settlers and Natives, around the residential school experience.

In the play I witnessed, a group of actors performed a short play, less than an hour with three separate but related scenes. Then the play was repeated. At various key points the director stopped the action and asked for volunteers from the audience to take the place of one or more of the actors on stage. With this new cast the scene was repeated. At the end of the scene the audience member returned to his/her place. The play continued on to another scene and the process was repeated. Later the audience as a whole and the actors were asked to share their thoughts on the play and its topic.

The situations and the characters depicted were more archetypal rather than individual which is why an audience member who had some thoughts on the situation portrayed could slip so easily into the vacated role. The people directing the event were traditionally trained theater people who seemed to have little or no knowledge of the sacred, so it was also done on a raised stage with the audience sitting out front.

Where possible I think a "theater in the round" layout would have been a better way to present this type of production, so the audience could have participated more freely. (I was one of those who would have liked to participate but couldn't due to where I was sitting, and my physical limitations, not able to climb on that stage.) However, conditions in the real world aren't always ideal. This was also a two to three hour event, (like a regular theater performance), but many people had much more to say on the topic, so a whole day workshop might be a better way to go when planning such an event.

I found this to be a powerful and enlightening experience and one perhaps I can use at some future time in my own work.

CHANNELING THE SACRED

Working with improvisation is very satisfying, because of its unpredictability. However, it is totally dependent on the power generated in the moment when it is performed. The other problem that comes up with improv in a ritual context is that, when an actor goes into channeling a divine persona, his or her sense of time totally changes. Once in persona, an actor must flow with the guidance being given. Problems may arise with other members in a ritual who are not being divinely directed, because they are expecting things to go as they were planned during the organizing sessions, and they don't always work that way.

Let me cite an example from a ceremonial in which the experienced dancers were to be abducted during the evening and taken away to the Underworld. (They had been told they had business with the Lady of the Underworld, but they did not know what that business was to be, or when it was to take place.) During the time they were gone, the new people would continue on, learning the dance steps to the yin and yang circles. Before our dance mistress began teaching them, I was to talk awhile (to give the actors time to create an Underworld and get into persona), and then we were supposed to have a demo by the old dancers so that the new people could see how the dance would look when it was put together the following night. When planning this, we estimated that we should give the group downstairs about 45 minutes to an hour to get ready.

What actually happened was that it took less time than expected, and once in persona, the servants of the Underworld were not about to be kept hanging around waiting for us to do everything we had said we were going to do when we planned all this. So, just after my talk, before we had time for the demo, we got invaded by very intimidating creatures from the Abyss who promptly seized all the experienced dancers and hustled them out of the room.

Unfortunately, this left our dance mistress holding the bag, so to speak. She coped quite well, but I'm sure she had a few moments of panic and frustration that things hadn't gone as planned. It is often hard for people who have not experienced channeling, or who are not in that altered state of consciousness at the time, to realize that the actors aren't deliberately trying to mess up by missing their cues; they are simply in another reality, and being guided by forces from outside themselves. When working in this way, people have to learn to be flexible and flow with the action, otherwise hurt feelings and frustrated communications are bound to arise.

While playing a role in sacred theatre, an actor may become the being he or she is enacting in the performance. This condition is a type of spiritual channeling, in which the actor's personality steps to one side (figuratively speaking), thus allowing his speech and actions to be directed by the Sacred Beings who have come to witness the ceremony, or the performance itself. After the channeling is over, the actor will probably be disoriented, and will not consciously remember much of what happened in the altered state. This inspired state may happen in the secular theatre as well, but is truly cultivated in places like Bali and India, where sacred dramas are still such a vital part of the spiritual life of the people.

In those cultures, this channeling process takes years of dedicated work to perfect. During that time, the actor-priests (both men and women) are carefully taught and supervised by experienced priests who act as their safety lines, never allowing the apprentices to go too far into the trance channeling experience. Over time, they learn their art so well that the skilled performers can make the stage come alive with the magic of the old myths.

In the theatrical traditions of Europe, occasionally there is a natural talent that can channel such power, but, for the most part, the theatre is secularized. It is rare to find someone trained and skilled in these ancient arts. This divine skill, however, is precisely what we are striving for as we develop and revive the community ceremonials of our past.

Sacred theatre is emerging once again out of the Dark Ages, but as yet the teachers of this ancient art are few and far between in Western culture. Performers trained in the secular theatre can adapt much of their training to serve the sacred theatre (which is why I recommend that my pupils take acting classes). Finding a teacher of sacred theatre is important if you can manage it, but if you cannot, I would offer a word of caution to take it slow, especially in areas like channeling, because the actor is so open and vulnerable to both good and evil influences. Before beginning any spiritual work, it is always wise to ground yourself and protect yourself with a sacred Circle or a protective talisman, thus allowing the energies to move through the body without causing harm.

What is usually meant by channeling is the type of psychic reading where the medium goes into trance and the client asks the spiritual beings channeled by the medium questions about his or her (the client's) life. This is what the Oracles at Delphi used to do. In improv, the actor-priests are channeling the Divine, but it's usually in the context of a story with a plot, rather than a divination.

The two (divination and improvisation) can be combined, to some extent. For example, in some of the rituals I have directed, the participants have gone into the Underworld and interacted with divinities channeled by the actors. The outline of the experience is scripted ahead of time, but the actual interaction is not, and the channeled divinities may choose to speak directly to some or all of the participants.

The question that always comes up when discussing this topic is, how can you tell when someone is truly channeling and when they are projecting their own "stuff," or, worse yet, using the Divine as a way of giving added authority to their own words and plans.

There is no hard and fast formula that I can give you to always tell what is "bull" and what is true. I can, however, offer a few suggestions that usually work. First of all, when on the receiving end of a channeled message from the Beyond, always trust your gut instinct. How does it feel to you? If it doesn't feel right, then either it isn't really channeled from the Gods, or else you may not be ready to accept what has been given to you at that time.

In either case, the wise course is to take such utterances with reservations. The trick here, of course, is to feel sufficiently confident in yourself that you won't feel guilty for not having enough "faith" to accept the message. Remember that, if it is a true sending, you can always ask that you be given that information again, in a way that you can better understand and accept.

On the other side of the coin, as the person doing the channeling, you have a sacred responsibility to always channel for the greatest good. This does not always mean sweetness and light; lessons can be harsh, but it does mean you have a duty to be aware that there are different energies out there, not all of them benevolent, and you must be aware of what you are opening up to and giving out. The more experience the actor-priest has, the less likely it is that his or her own personal "stuff" will get in the way of what is being transmitted.

Sensitive people say they can feel an energy presence enter the room when true channeling is being done. I would also suggest, if it is possible, to observe the person who does the channeling after the work is over. To channel means running a lot of very powerful energy through the body. Most channels are affected in some way by this process. Some may feel weak or be unable to talk while they are adjusting back to our physical reality. Symptoms vary, but it has been my observation that although people respond differently, all are affected in some way.

⚜

SACRED CLOWNING

In our modern secular theatre tradition, the character of the jester or trickster has almost been lost. Around the world, however, these sacred clowns still play an important role in the spiritual lives of their people through ceremony. In North America, there were Raven and Coyote and the Heyoka clowns. In Europe, there was the court jester or fool, who gave the king honesty and spoke the shadowed truth that no one else dared bring out in the light of day.

The Contraries, or clowns, in Native cultures brings humor to ceremony when their antics poke fun at the ridiculousness of everyday life. These Heyokas may dress funny, and walk and do everything backwards, but in spite of the laughter they are not a joke, but highly respected for their medicine power. As an anthropologist once told me, clowns reflect the chaotic elements of their community's psyche that if expressed at other times and in other ways, would destroy the fabric of the group.

This sounds very scientific and I, for one, had not thought of the trickster's role in quite those terms, but it is true that clowns can act crazy and are usually given free license to do just about whatever they please during Native ceremonies. It is recognized by the other medicine elders that, in the seeming irreverence of the clown's words and actions, there is great honesty and thus great spiritual wisdom. Those who know, try not to anger the Contraries, because their lessons, having that trickster element, are often harsh and not gentle in their messages.

Throughout the ages, the trickster, in any culture, has been both honored and feared. Little children, especially, recognize that clowns can be scary as well as funny. Like certain aspects of the Underworld Goddesses, the clowns gain much of their power from their link with the unconscious. This may manifest in frightening masked figures who punish wrongs and abduct people, or in less terrifying beings like the Hopi thought police who slap paint across the faces of anyone having unpleasant or distracting thoughts at a ceremony, thus using ridicule as a means of control.

Modern secular clowns who I have talked to about their training tell me that the development of their clown personas included journeys into the Underworld, or their own unconscious to gather materials for what would eventually become their clown characters. In this sense, their training is very similar to that undertaken by sacred clowns in other cultures, and probably comes down in a direct line of descent from the training of medieval jesters and fools.

What I know about clowning I know more by instinct than by instruction, but it is a powerful tool in ceremony as long as the trickster is treated with respect. When inviting the trickster to a ceremony, be prepared for the unexpected. Anything can happen, and usually does. I'll never forget the time a big wind that harmed nothing else blew the door of the hall we were dancing in off the frame, after we had invited the trickster to our rite. (Some of us really sweated blood trying to get that fixed before the owners saw it.)

I strongly believe that the sacred clowns have a place in our community ceremonial systems, just as they did of old, but we need to take special care when working with this most powerful energy. As with any kind of channeling of the Divine, there is a fine line between working with sacred energy and projecting personal ego trips. When channeled by an experienced adept, trickster energy can teach many hard-to-learn lessons. When done without the guidance of the Sacred Ones, however, it can be incredibly painful and cruel.

Even today in the secular theatre, clowning is a little-known and somewhat secretive art. Instruction in its techniques may take some search. I found that out when doing research on clowning for this part of the book. There doesn't seem to be much written down about the actual teaching of the art. All I could find were the usual anthropologists' descriptions of clowning witnessed in other cultures around the world. This is very refreshing to me, because, although it was frustrating for this book's research, it tells me that much of the ancient knowledge of this tradition may still be intact, and there if you have the patience to seek it out. Since there are still clowns in the world, their skill must still be passed on privately from teacher to student, as it has been from time immemorial.

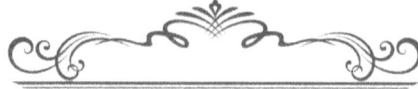

Some Further Thoughts

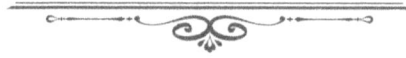

Most sacred theatre that I know of in the modern Pagan communities relies on a memorized or read script. This scripted drama works only if the actor-priests have taken enough time to fluently learn their lines before the ritual. When everyone is nervous and has only a day or two to practice (if that), little power can be raised or focused, because the spirit just can't come through all those blocked channels.

Let me go back a bit, and talk more about the style of performance that is most appropriate for the ritual theatre. The older style of "theatre in the round" is much better than a performance on a raised stage. For a theatre in the round performance, I suggest having a narrator who will explain to the audience any background or other material they will need to know. I also suggest the use of a chorus that chants from time to time, and that carries on a low, rhythmic drumbeat as a background drone throughout the entire performance. (Please, if possible, don't play a tape for this!) The background drone acts as a relaxer to the older centres of the brain, thus inviting a light trance state in which to experience the performance.

The actors themselves should wear masks or half-masks and be skilled at expressing themselves through movement, because much of the story will be acted out in mime and dance, rather than long memorized dialogue. If the number of players is small, actors and chorus members can interchange roles at various parts of the production. Other musical instruments and props can be added, and impressive-looking costumes for all are a real must.

The aim is to convey, through the actors' performance, real feelings and experiences. All depends on the artists' skill, because in order for the play to be performed wherever a ritual is taking place, the set must be very simple and very portable.

In certain plays, there may be a strict separation between audience and actors, while at other times there may be some interaction between the two. Sometimes there will be no human audience at all, only players in the divine drama. Each of these three styles works well in the ceremonial context, if the participants are able to let go of their inhibitions and allow their imagination and creativity to flow freely in this spirit of serious play.

To help with the feeling and creativity of your work, I would suggest holding one or more short rituals to dedicate the actors and their gear to the service of the deities who you want to call upon in your performances. A dedication ceremony is like a statement of intent. The ritual makes it very clear to both human and deity what the purpose of your art will be. It can also add personal integrity and commitment to the plays and performances you undertake. Each performance should be viewed as an offering to the Sacred, and the actors should proceed with that in mind.

The field of sacred theatre is a large and complex one, in which I feel very much the beginner, but I hope my comments will inspire other persons and groups to study theatre in other cultures and experiment with how it can become a powerful part of the living spiritual traditions of our own time.

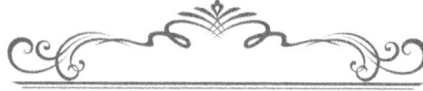

Conclusion

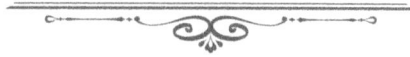

This book is a compilation of many years study and work. Rereading the manuscript after several years in which I went on to other projects that didn't include working much with large group rituals, I gained the time and space to re-examine this book and its contents with fresh eyes. To my surprise, the work hadn't gone out of date, and there wasn't much I wished to add or change in this new edition. (Except for a few typos missed in the earlier editing process.)

As I've said before in these pages it is possible to rediscover and create a vibrant and workable spiritual model to guide us through the difficult times ahead. For some that path is easier, because there are still functioning systems kept safe and passed down from our ancestors to the present to give us a base on which to build for the future. But these teachings aren't enough by themselves. We who are living now, and those who follow us must understand at a deep level the essence behind the form of a religious practice. And to do this, I believe, will take time and personal commitment, not only by the individual, but the community in which these individuals live.

Prayer, personal study, finding guides and teachers to help us along our path is all part of the process we chose when agreeing to be born into this physical world. It is my wish that this book will be just one more guide along the reader's way. This book, as with other books I have written, is my legacy to the future. Its content is offered with love and the hope that it can be of some use to all people around the world, including my biological and adopted descendants.

Dear Reader, you have been born into a time of great change in a very troubled world. I believe that ceremony has a place in helping to mold the future for the Greater Good of all living beings, and it is with that hope that I offer this book.

Celu Amberstone (Cornwoman)

Don't miss out!

Visit the website below and you can sign up to receive emails whenever Celu Amberstone publishes a new book. There's no charge and no obligation.

https://books2read.com/r/B-A-YGQM-CVQSB

BOOKS 2 READ

Connecting independent readers to independent writers.

Did you love *Deepening the Power: Community Ritual and Sacred Theatre*? Then you should read *Blessings of the Blood: A Book of Menstrual Lore and Rituals for Women*[1] by Celu Amberstone!

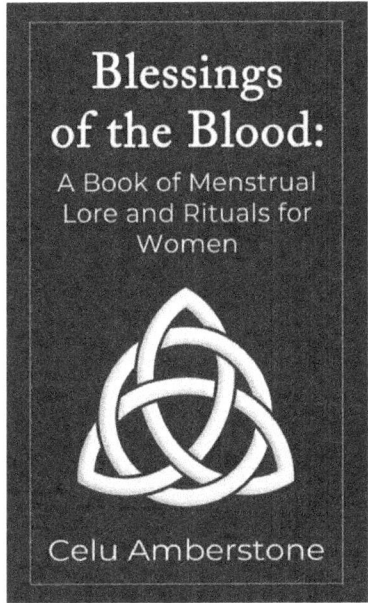

"I have heard a call across a million years. I will answer it."

Here is a book of women's rituals surrounding and embracing menstruation. With sensitivity, author Celu Amberstone gathers prayers and spiritual experiences from women celebrating their bodies and their profoundly personal experiences. Readers looking to support personal identity and strengthen a sense of community will find much of interest in *Blessings of the Blood: a Book of Menstrual Lore and Rituals for Women*.

"May the works of your hands and the meditations of your heart be healing."

This edition is a new release of a celebrated book previously released in 1991 from Beach Holme Press. For years, readers eagerly sought the book through used book dealers. Celu Amberstone and Kashallan Press are proud to release this new edition by popular request. *Blessings of the Blood* is available

---

1. https://books2read.com/u/mB25QO

2. https://books2read.com/u/mB25QO

in an affordable ebook version for the first time, to complement the handsome trade paperback.

For anyone interested in possibly feeling better about their blood, I highly recommend the book "Blessings Of The Blood" By Celu Amberstone. It is a wonderful book with personal stories of menarche, menopause and creativeness. It really opened my eyes to just how sacred and beautiful our blood is.

-review on Mum website

This is one of the best books on the subject of menstruation, and I wish they would reissue Celu's masterpiece! Filled with anecdotes, storytelling and empathy.

-SMB, review on Amazon

Also by Celu Amberstone

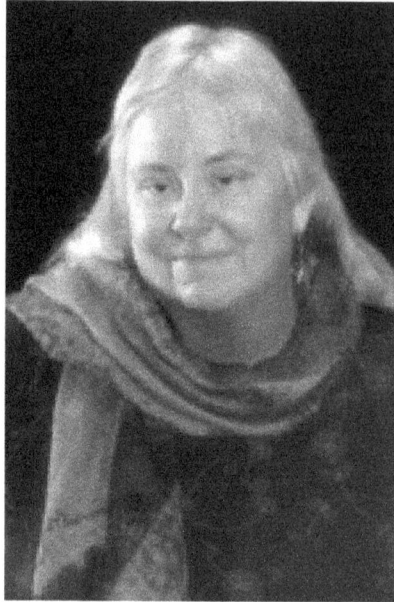

About the Author

Celu is of mixed Cherokee and Scots-Irish ancestry. Celu Amberstone was one of the few young people in her family to take an interest in learning Traditional Native crafts and medicine ways. This interest made several of the older members of her family very happy while annoying others.

Legally blind since birth, she has defied her limitations and spent much of her life avoiding cities. Moving to Canada after falling in love with a Métis-Cree man from Manitoba, she has lived in the rain forests of the west coast, a tepee in the desert and a small village in Canada's arctic. Along the way she also managed to acquire a BA in cultural anthropology and an MA in health education. Celu loves telling stories and reading. She lives in Victoria British Columbia near her grown children and grandchildren.

About the Publisher

Kashallan Press is an independent publisher releasing books by author Celu Amberstone. Among her books are critically-acclaimed works now re-released by Kashallan Press, and new works showcasing her talents in writing both fiction and non-fiction.

www.ingramcontent.com/pod-product-compliance
Lightning Source LLC
LaVergne TN
LVHW011327080426
835513LV00006B/232